DR. SAROJ PACHAURI, MD, PhD, DPH, DR. ASH PACHAURI, PhD, DRISHYA PATHAK

Public Health Uncoded with Dr. Saroj Pachauri

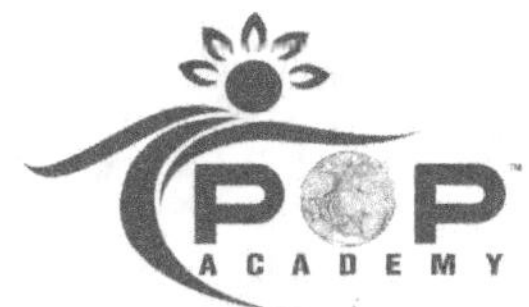

Contents

Foreword   vi

Acknowledgement   ix

INTRODUCTION AND RATIONALE   1

PART 1: SEXUAL AND REPRODUCTIVE HEALTH
AND RIGHTS   2

PODCAST 1: SEXUAL AND REPRODUCTIVE HEALTH   3

John Townsend   5

Summary of the Podcast   8

What are Sexual and Reproductive Health and Rights (SRHR)?   10

PODCAST 2: MATERNAL HEALTH   14

Aparajita Gogoi   16

Summary of the Podcast   19

What is maternal health?   21

PODCAST 3: SAFE ABORTION   24

Beverly Winikoff   26

Summary of the Podcast   29

What is safe abortion?   31

PODCAST 4: HIV & AIDS   34

Rajiv Dua   36

Summary of the podcast   39

What are HIV and AIDS?   42

PODCAST 5: GENDER   45

Madhu Bala Nath   47

Summary of the podcast   50

What is gender?   52

PODCAST 6: HEALTH COMMUNICATION   55

Anjali Nayyar   57

Summary of the podcast   60

What is health communication?   62

PART 2: CHILD HEALTH   65

PODCAST 7: CHILDHOOD OBESITY   66

Seema Chandra   68

Summary of the podcast   71

What is childhood obesity?   73

PODCAST 8: THE IMPACT OF CLIMATE CHANGE ON CHILD HEALTH   76

Karina Weinstein   78

Summary of the podcast   81

What are the impacts of climate change on child health?   83

PART 3: HEALTH IMPACTS OF CLIMATE CHANGE   87

PODCAST 9: IMPACT OF CLIMATE CHANGE ON HUMAN HEALTH   88

Antonio Sarmiento Galán   90

Summary of the podcast   93

What are the impacts of climate change on human health?   96

PODCAST 10: SARGASSUM, A BROWN SEAWEED   100

Norma Patricia Muñoz Sevilla   102

Summary of the podcast   105

What is sargassum and how does it affect human health?   107

PODCAST 11: IMPACTS OF PERSISTENT ORGANIC POLLUTANTS AND...   110

Girija Bharat   112

Summary of the podcast   115

What are Persistent organic pollutants (POPs)?   118

PODCAST 12: THE COVID-19 PANDEMIC   122

Bulbul Sood   124

Summary of the podcast   127

What is COVID-19 and what are its Impacts on Health?   129

PODCAST 13: PUBLIC HEALTH ENTREPRENEURSHIP   133

Quisha Umemba   134

Summary of the Podcast   137

What is public health entrepreneurship?   140

PODCAST 14: NAVIGATING THE INTERSECTION OF WATER, CLIMATE...   144

Debadutta Parija   146

Summary of the podcast   149

What are the intersections between water, climate, and...   151

AUTHORS' BIOS   155

LIST OF ACRONYMS   164

RESOURCE LIST   167

REFERENCES   172

Foreword

East or west, rural or urban, rich or poor, diagnosis or treatment, genuine knowledge of public health is a compelling necessity in today's world of information and misinformation. In order to counteract misinformation and promote health, public health experts and scholars must guide us. After all, the purpose of life is to lead a life of purpose.

Dr. Saroj Pachauri has succinctly and passionately embraced the new podcast platform. She has undertaken discussion and dialogue with highly experienced experts and scholars in public health to guide and engage the public by presenting research results in ways that can be understood and, more importantly, implemented by expert-guided methods as solutions. The book you hold compels you to turn the pages, knowing that you are in safe hands and that public health experts are guiding you. Public health experts, through their special expertise and extensive experience, provide deep insights into problems through research and suggest creative ways to address them. This book provides podcast discussions on various topics, including sexual and reproductive health and rights, child health, and the health impacts of climate change. The good news is that the plan is to continue these podcasts to foster a culture of assessing and creatively addressing public health problems. The audience for these podcast discussions includes policy planners, health advocates, public health professionals, research scientists, and climate scientists. The aim is to promote the health of individuals and communities.

By Prof. Sneh Bhargava, MD

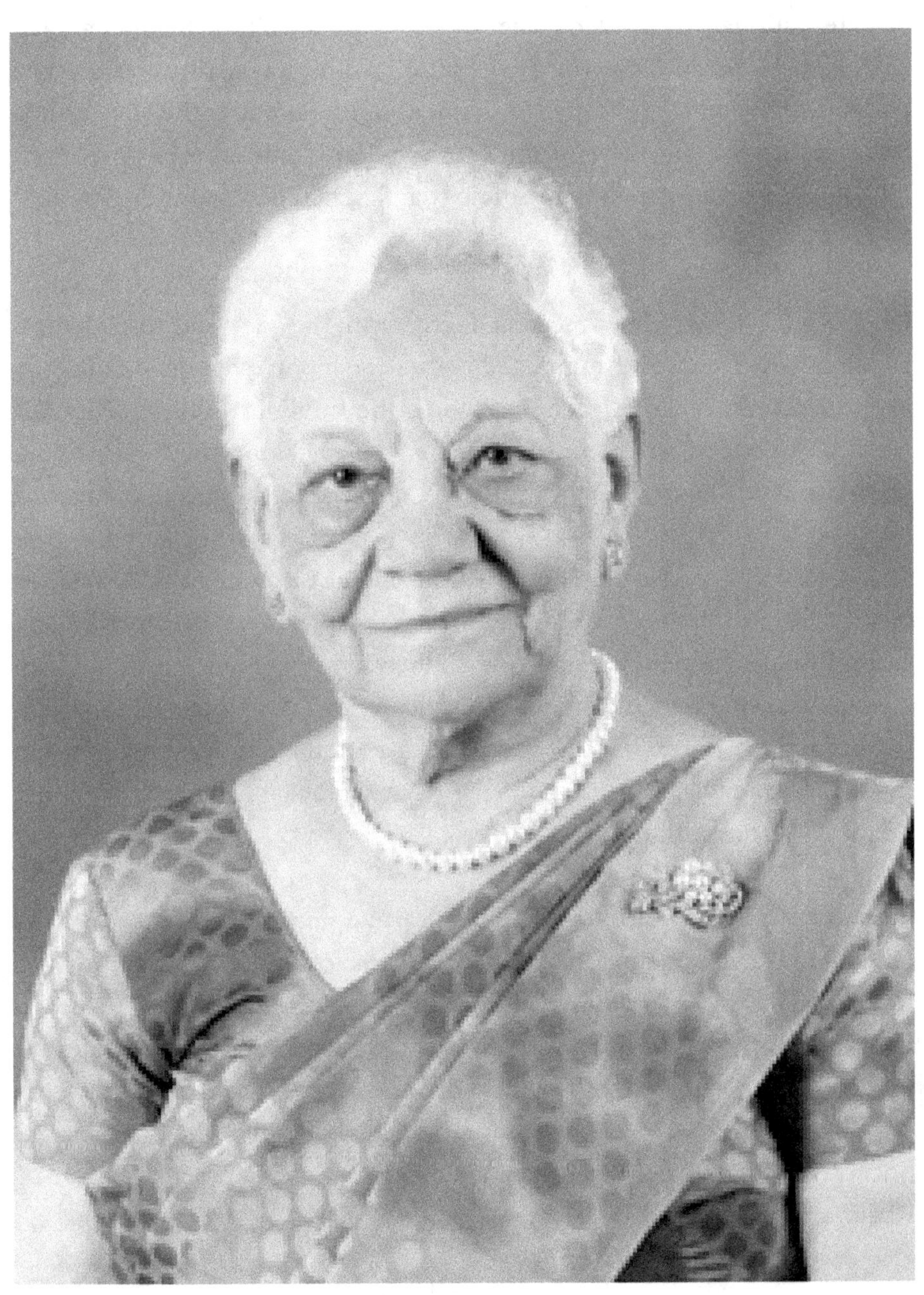

Dr. Sneh Bhargava

An internationally respected leader in radiology education, Sneh Bhargava, MD, is the Medical Director of the Sitaram Bhartia Institute of Science and Research and chair of the Department of Radiology at the Dharmshila Narayan Super Specialty Hospital, both in New Delhi. She is a professor emeritus of the Department of Radiology at the All India Institute of Medical Sciences (AIIMS), New Delhi.

Dr. Bhargava received her medical degree from the Lady Harding Medical College, New Delhi, and completed her fellowship in diagnostic radiology at the Westminster Medical School (now the Imperial College School of Medicine), London. She returned to India with a Diploma in Medical Radio Diagnosis (DMRD) awarded by the Royal College of Physicians and Surgeons.

She was the first female director of AIIMS and the only one in its 70 years of history; Dr. Bhargava helped to establish the departments of neuroradiology, cardiovascular radiology, pediatric radiology, and interventional radiology. She established the Medical Education Technology Center at AIIMS, which is designed to offer medical students information about learning to teach medicine. She was also a part of the team that established the National Medical Journal of India.

Former president of the Indian Radiological and Imaging Association (IRIA), Dr. Bhargava was chair of several committees for the Medical Council of India. She has received numerous lifetime achievement awards, including the Millennium Award 2000 from IRIA. For her distinguished contributions to medicine, she received the Padma Shri, one of the highest civilian awards in India. She also received the Honorable Membership of the Radiological Society of North America and the Fellowship of the American College of Radiology.

Acknowledgement

We extend our heartfelt gratitude to all the public health experts whose voices enriched "Public Health Uncoded with Dr. Saroj Pachauri." Special thanks to the authors, the technical team behind the podcast development, including the music composer and post-production team, for their invaluable contributions.

Public Health Uncoded with Dr. Saroj Pachauri

Dr. Saroj Pachauri, a public health expert, provides commentary on some of the major public health problems of the times. She discusses how the determinants of public health are at play, especially in high-risk and vulnerable groups. Every month, Dr. Saroj Pachauri, a doctor of medicine and a distinguished public health scholar with over 60 years of experience, unpacks key public health concerns and opportunities in the current global arena with evidence and insights.

Drishya Pathak is a researcher who hosts the public health uncoded podcast. She has also been a research associate and POP Youth mentor with POP (Protect Our Planet) Movement for six years.

Music composition by Edgar Andres Martínez Lozano, POP Movement's Music Ambassador.

Technical and post-production by Manish Gupta, POP Movement's creative Youth Mentor.

INTRODUCTION AND RATIONALE

The podcast series "Public Health Uncoded" is designed to stimulate discussion on important public health issues. Discussions are undertaken with public health experts who provide important insights into the problems and discuss how these problems can be resolved. These professionals illuminate the issues through their extensive experience and special expertise and suggest ways to address them.

The field of public health is vast and continually evolving. Current problems must be addressed, and new ones that emerge continuously need redressal. The experts interviewed suggest innovative strategies for addressing these public health problems. The rise of new communication channels, alongside traditional media, has created a breeding ground for misinformation. To counter this, the scientific community needs to embrace new platforms such as podcasts to actively engage the public by presenting research results in easily understood ways. This discourse with the experts in the field is an important resource, and it is shared with a broad audience that listens to the podcasts. Your role as part of this audience is crucial, as the information is disseminated widely, and your engagement is key to addressing these public health issues.

The plan is to continue these podcasts to address public health issues as they arise, and thereby foster a culture of assessing and creatively addressing public health problems. This ongoing conversation includes you, the listener, as an integral part of the process.

PART 1: SEXUAL AND REPRODUCTIVE HEALTH AND RIGHTS

The podcasts in this book are organized according to the topics they cover. The first section features six significant discussions on Sexual and Reproductive Health and Rights (SRHR).

Sexual and Reproductive Health and Rights is a critically important theme. It includes women's health, maternal health, family planning, abortion, and HIV/AIDS. Gender cuts across all these issues within SRHR. There is an ongoing need to research to understand the problems, their causes, and outcomes, and to design programs based on research evidence to prevent these problems and to develop strategies for implementing programs in different contexts, targeting services to various client groups, and developing policy frameworks to guide the implementation of programs to address SRHR problems.

The podcasts included within this theme would interest policy-makers, research scientists, service providers in the public and private sectors, and the users of services, especially women.

PODCAST 1: SEXUAL AND REPRODUCTIVE HEALTH

Sexual and Reproductive Health (SRH) is an important area that needs to be urgently addressed. The problem of HIV & AIDS falls within the area of sexual health. Maternal health, family planning, and abortion are included under the umbrella of reproductive health. Reproductive health technologies, in particular contraceptive technologies including intra-uterine devices (IUDs), oral contraceptive pills, contraceptive implants, female sterilization, and vasectomy, play an essential role in sexual and reproductive health. Contraceptive choices for women and women's autonomy are important, as are the role of men in contraceptive use and in supporting women's choices and the use of contraceptive methods for spacing and limiting births.

Pregnancies that are too early, too late, or too closely spaced are risky. The ideal age to have children is 20 to 30, but that depends on personal preferences. Global trends show that the average number of children per family has been decreasing over time.

The audience for this podcast includes research scientists, policy planners, service providers, and users of services, especially women.

Questions addressed

1) What is the origin of the concept of sexual and reproductive rights?

2) How can families and communities address the sexual and reproductive health information needs of young people?

3) What is the importance of avoiding pregnancies that are too soon, too late, or too close together?

4) What is the difference between spacing and limiting births?

5) What is the role of men in pregnancy planning?

6) What contraceptives are suitable to different clients?

Keywords

Sexual and reproductive health and rights, population control, fertility control, maternal and infant mortality, contraceptive methods, and infertility

John Townsend

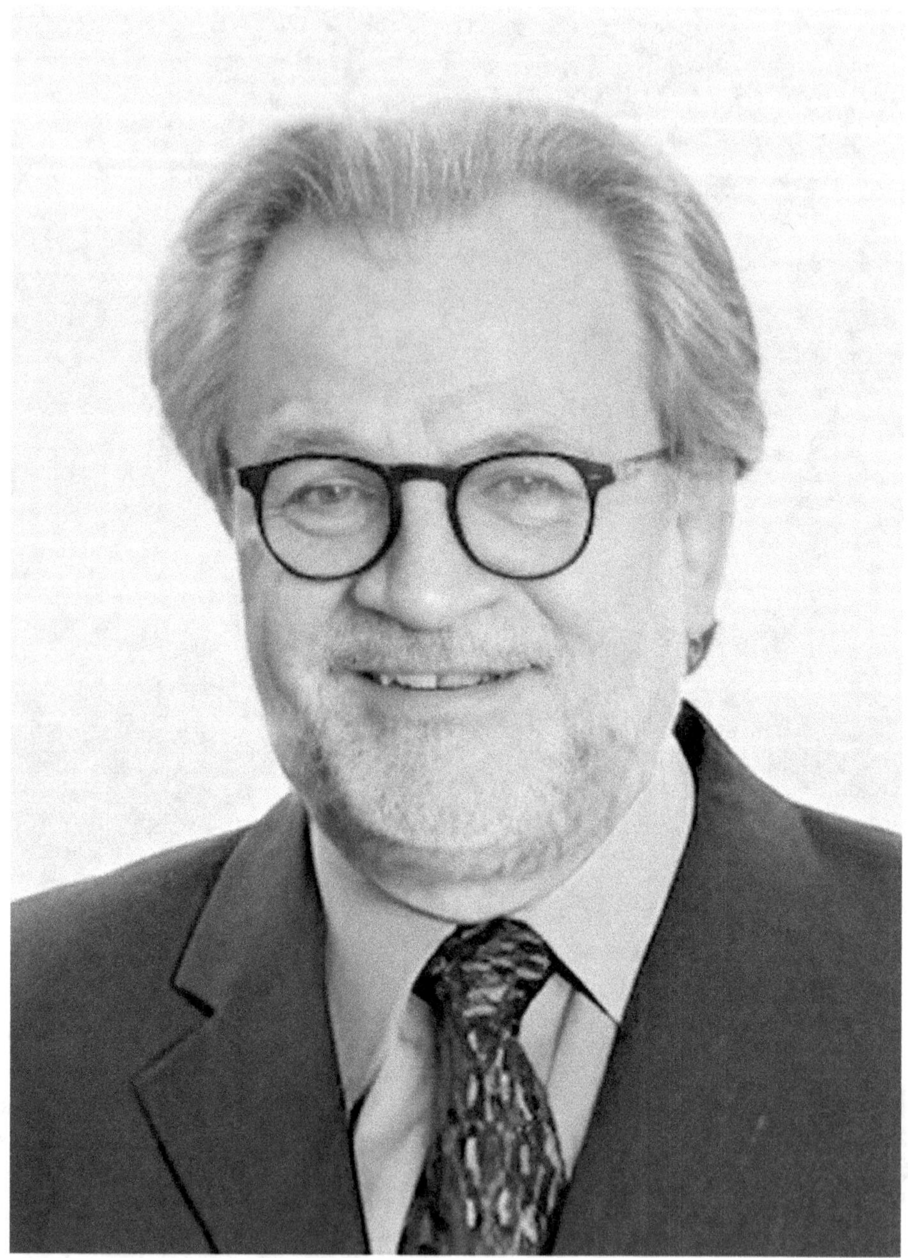

Dr. John Townsend, Chair, Rotary Action Group for Reproductive, Maternal and Child Health, and Chair, Ethical Review Board (IRB), International Center for Research on Women

D r. John W Townsend is a highly accomplished expert in the field of reproductive health and maternal and child health. He has held various leadership positions at the Population Council including Director of Reproductive Health and Director of Country Strategy. He focused on policy development and on designing interventions to improve reproductive health service delivery systems with a particular emphasis on client rights. Dr. Townsend is currently working with the Rotary Action Group for Reproductive, Maternal, and Child Health. He serves as Chair of the Reproductive Health Supplies Coalition and of the Institutional Review Board of the International Center for Research on Women. He has been involved in numerous advisory boards and task forces related to reproductive health and has been a reviewer for several peer-reviewed journals. Dr. Townsend has extensive international experience, having worked and traveled in over 35 countries. He holds a PhD in social psychology and has received multiple awards for his research and contributions to the field of reproductive health.

Summary of the Podcast

In this episode of Public Health Uncoded, Dr. Saroj Pachauri and our guest Dr. John Townsend, a reproductive health specialist, delved into the topic of sexual and reproductive health and rights.

In their conversation they covered a range of issues related to reproductive health and family planning. They began the discussion by focusing on the needs and desires of individuals, particularly young women, and the ethical considerations surrounding reproductive technologies (1).

The conversation then moved on to statistics related to births and pregnancies, which highlighted the risks associated with early and late pregnancies. Dr. John Townsend cited facts and analytical points on pregnancies before the age of 20 that have a higher risk of mortality. Pregnancies after the age of 35 come with their own set of challenges.

The ideal time to have a child is between the ages of 20 and 30, but individual choices may vary. The importance of spacing pregnancies with a gap of two to three years was emphasized to ensure optimal child development and allow women to pursue other roles beyond motherhood (2).

Different methods of contraception for spacing and limiting births were discussed. These included intrauterine devices, contraceptive implants, female sterilization, and vasectomy. Dr. Townsend emphasized the role of men in contraceptive use and in supporting women's choices.

The conversation also touched on global population trends, including the decreasing average number of children per family. Certain groups raised concerns about labor availability. Dr. Townsend argued against coercion and stressed the importance of individual autonomy in reproductive decision-making.

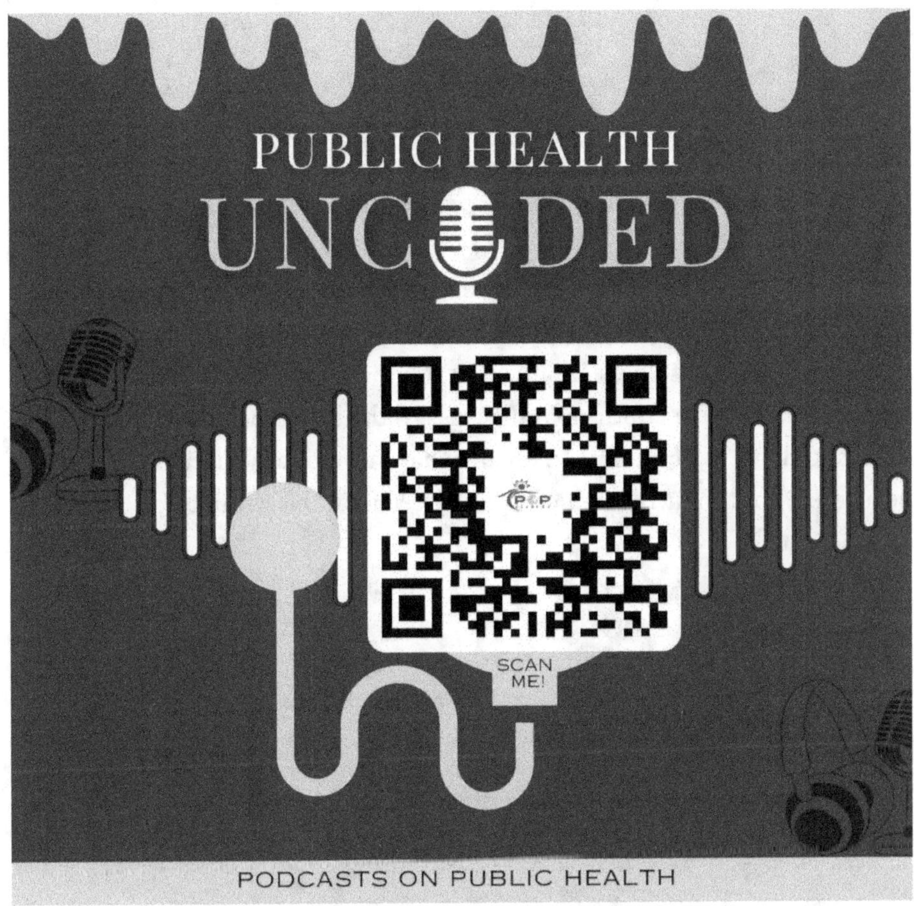

Scan the QR Code or follow the link to listen
https://thepopmovement.org/podcast-public-health-uncoded/

What are Sexual and Reproductive Health and Rights (SRHR)?

What are Sexual and Reproductive Health and Rights?

Sexual and Reproductive Health and Rights (SRHR) encompass a wide range of issues related to sexuality and reproduction, including the right to have a safe and satisfying sex life, the right to decide if and when to have children and access to the necessary information and means to do so. SRHR aims to ensure that individuals can make informed decisions about their reproductive lives free from discrimination, coercion, and violence.

Key Components of SRHR

Sexual Health:

A state of physical, emotional, mental, and social wellbeing in relation to sexuality.

Positive and respectful approach to sexuality and sexual relationships.

Possibility of having pleasurable and safe sexual experiences, free of coercion, discrimination, and violence.

Reproductive Health:

A state of complete physical, mental, and social wellbeing in all matters relating to the reproductive system.

Ability to have a responsible, satisfying, and safe sex life.

Capability to reproduce and the freedom to decide if, when, and how often to do so.

Reproductive Rights:

The fundamental rights of all couples and individuals to decide freely and responsibly the number, spacing, and timing of their children.

Right to attain the highest standard of sexual and reproductive health.

Right to make decisions concerning reproduction free of discrimination, coercion, and violence.

Access to Services:

Ensuring that individuals have access to appropriate healthcare services, including family planning, contraception, maternal healthcare, and safe abortion services.

Comprehensive sexual education to make informed choices.

Elimination of Violence:

Addressing and eliminating gender-based violence, sexual abuse, and harmful practices like female genital mutilation (FGM) and child marriage.

References

World Health Organization (WHO):

WHO offers extensive resources on sexual and reproductive health, emphasizing the importance of comprehensive SRHR services and education. For more details, visit WHO's SRHR Page.

United Nations Population Fund (UNFPA):

UNFPA focuses on promoting reproductive health and rights, providing resources and advocacy for family planning, maternal health, and the prevention of gender-based violence. Learn more at UNFPA's SRHR Page.

Guttmacher Institute:

The Guttmacher Institute conducts research and policy analysis on sexual and reproductive health and rights, offering valuable data and insights into global SRHR trends and issues. Explore their resources at Guttmacher Institute.

Centers for Disease Control and Prevention (CDC):

The CDC provides guidelines, resources, and research on reproductive health, including contraception, maternal health, and prevention of sexually transmitted infections (STIs). Visit CDC's Reproductive Health Page.

International Planned Parenthood Federation (IPPF):

IPPF works globally to ensure access to sexual and reproductive health services and rights. They offer resources and advocacy tools on SRHR. Visit IPPF's SRHR Page.

Ensuring comprehensive SRHR services is crucial for promoting overall health, gender equality, and sustainable development.

PODCAST 2: MATERNAL HEALTH

Maternal health is related to women's health before, during, and after pregnancy. The problems of maternal mortality and morbidity need to be urgently addressed, especially in developing countries where the rates of maternal mortality and morbidity are high. Maternal health has deep connections with gender disparity, gender-power dynamics, and the challenges women and girls face in accessing services.

There is a need to develop comprehensive approaches to address social norms, health infrastructure, and the empowerment of women. Investing in the health workforce, promoting respectful maternity care, and adopting a holistic intersectoral approach to develop program strategies for improving maternal health is important. There is an urgent need to amplify women's voices and include them in decision-making to ensure that programs address their needs.

This podcast discussion focused on India. This information would be useful for public health professionals, women advocates, policy planners, service providers, and service users, especially women.

Questions addressed

1. What is the maternal health situation in India? What have been the major gains in recent years, and what are the reasons for gaps in progress?

2. What is the role of healthcare providers and of women and families to promote safe motherhood?
3. What strategies can help India deliver maternal healthcare to the last mile?
4. What are the priorities for addressing maternal health issues as we move forward?

Keywords

Maternal health, gender equity, empowerment, quality of care, institutional delivery, and health workforce

Aparajita Gogoi

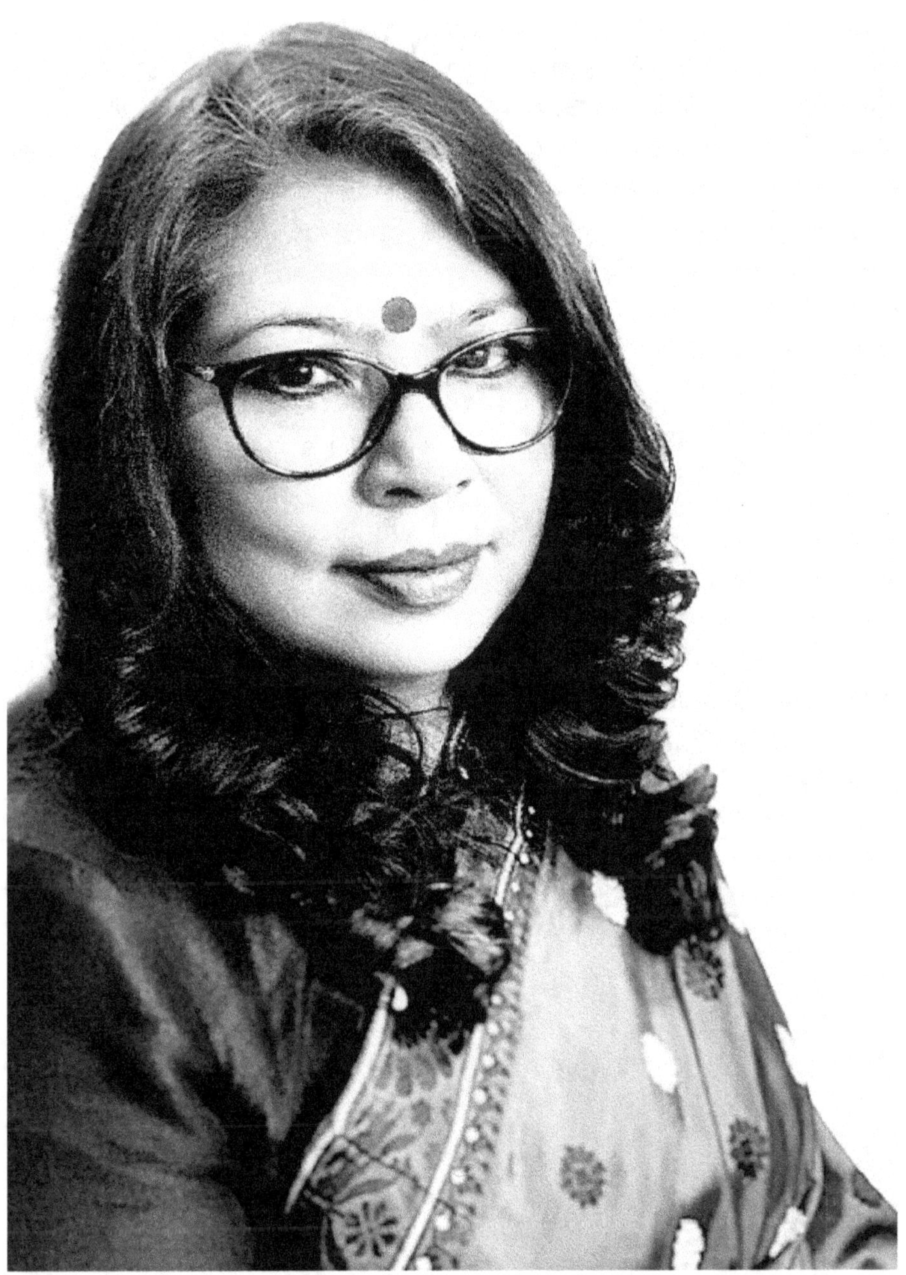

Dr. Aparajita Gogoi, Executive Director, Center for Catalyzing Change

Dr. Aparajita Gogoi serves as Executive Director, Centre for Catalyzing Change, a nonprofit that supports women and girl's access, rights, and equity. It is dedicated to creating lasting systems change at the grassroots working with adolescent girls and women by leveraging existing platforms to provide sustainable solutions.

Dr. Gogoi is also the National Coordinator of the White Ribbon Alliance for Safe Motherhood in India. Under her leadership, the very successful Whatwomenwant campaign was conceived and implemented in India. She also guided the global Whatwomenwant campaign as the global co-chair.

She holds a PhD degree in international politics from the Jawaharlal Nehru University, New Delhi,

On 8th March 2011, the Guardian, U.K, marked International Women's Day by selecting 100 of world's most inspiring women. Aparajita Gogoi was named as one of these 100 women. India Today, India's premier magazine, featured her as an Unsung Hero in its Anniversary Issue in December 2019.

Summary of the Podcast

In this podcast of Public Health Uncoded, Dr. Saroj Pachauri invited Dr. Aparajita Gogoi, an expert on maternal health. Dr. Gogoi contributed a chapter 'Claiming as equals: Journey of women leaders' and 'Respectful maternity care: A cornerstone for improving maternal health' in the book entitled 'Transforming Unequal Gender Relations in India and Beyond: An Intersectional Perspective on Challenges and Opportunities' edited by Dr. Saroj Pachauri and Dr. Ravi Verma (3).

In this podcast of Public Health Uncoded, Dr. Saroj Pachauri and Dr. Aparajita Gogoi examined the multifaceted issues related to maternal health, highlighting its deep connection to gender discrimination and societal norms. Dr. Gogoi discussed the challenges women face in accessing quality healthcare and the importance of addressing gender-based power dynamics to improve maternal health outcomes (4). She said that despite the global progress made in reducing maternal mortality, recent data indicate a troubling stagnation in it's progress in India. She emphasized the need for renewed efforts to address this problem. Successful strategies implemented in countries like India were discussed. The importance of comprehensive approaches that address social norms, healthcare infrastructure, and women empowerment was emphasized.

Recommendations made by Dr. Gogoi included investing in the health workforce, promoting respectful maternity care, and adopting a holistic, intersectoral approach to maternal health (5)(6). Central to these recommendations was the imperative to amplify women's voices and involve women in decision-making processes to ensure that programs were designed and implemented with their needs and preferences in mind.

Scan the QR Code or follow the link to listen
https://thepopmovement.org/podcast-public-health-uncoded/

What is maternal health?

What is maternal health?

Maternal health refers to women's health during pregnancy, childbirth, and postpartum. Ensuring maternal health is critical for mothers' and babies' wellbeing. Key components of maternal health include:

Antenatal Care: Regular medical check-ups, screenings, and interventions during pregnancy to monitor and promote the health of the mother and the developing fetus.

Safe Delivery Practices: Ensuring that childbirth is attended by skilled healthcare providers who can manage normal deliveries and handle complications that may arise during labor and delivery.

Postpartum Care: Health care is provided to the mother and her newborn immediately after birth and during the first six weeks postpartum to address complications and promote recovery.

Access to Health Services: Ensuring women access necessary health services, including family planning, to prevent unintended pregnancies and space births for optimal health outcomes.

Education and Support: Education on nutrition, breastfeeding, newborn care, and recognizing danger signs during pregnancy and childbirth.

References

World Health Organization (WHO):

WHO provides comprehensive guidelines and resources on maternal health, emphasizing the importance of quality care before, during, and after childbirth. For more details, visit WHO's Maternal Health Overview.

United Nations Population Fund (UNFPA):

UNFPA promotes maternal health and ensures safe childbirth through various programs and initiatives. For more information, check UNFPA's Maternal Health Page.

Centers for Disease Control and Prevention (CDC):

CDC provides resources, research, and guidelines on maternal health, including strategies to prevent maternal mortality and improve health outcomes for mothers and infants. Learn more at CDC's Maternal and Infant Health Page.

March of Dimes:

This organization works to improve the health of mothers and babies by preventing birth defects, premature birth, and infant mortality. They offer extensive resources on maternal health. Visit March of Dimes' Maternal Health Resources.

Guttmacher Institute:

The Guttmacher Institute conducts research and policy analysis on maternal health, providing valuable insights into global trends and issues. Explore their resources at Guttmacher Institute's Maternal Health Section.

Ensuring comprehensive maternal health care reduces maternal and neonatal mortality and promotes healthy families and communities.

PODCAST 3: SAFE ABORTION

The need for providing abortion services cannot be overstated. Women will always have unwanted pregnancies so there is clear need to ensure that they have access to safe abortion services. Surgical abortion requires a health infrastructure with trained physicians who can conduct surgical abortions. With the availability of medical abortion in recent years, it is now possible for women to take a pill, mifepristone, and have a safe abortion at home. Safe medical abortion during the first trimester has become a reality for women in developed and developing countries.

Abortion, however, is a politically charged issue. In the USA, for example, where mifepristone can be obtained online, women can now safely undergo abortion at home. However, pro-life forces have resulted in abortion bans in several states.

Legal and political factors affect the provision of abortion services. Women's power and autonomy, reproductive choice, and the availability of online abortion services are also important.

This information would interest legal experts, policy planners, women advocates, service providers, and users of services, especially women.

Questions addressed

1. Do all women worldwide have access to safe and effective abortion?

2. Who is allowed to provide abortion?
3. Can you have an abortion with a pill alone using no instruments?
4. What has been the impact of the wide availability of abortion pills?
5. What other new technologies might be available in the foreseeable future?

Keywords

Safe abortion, legalization, medical access, pills for abortion, political dimensions, and cultural norms

Beverly Winikoff

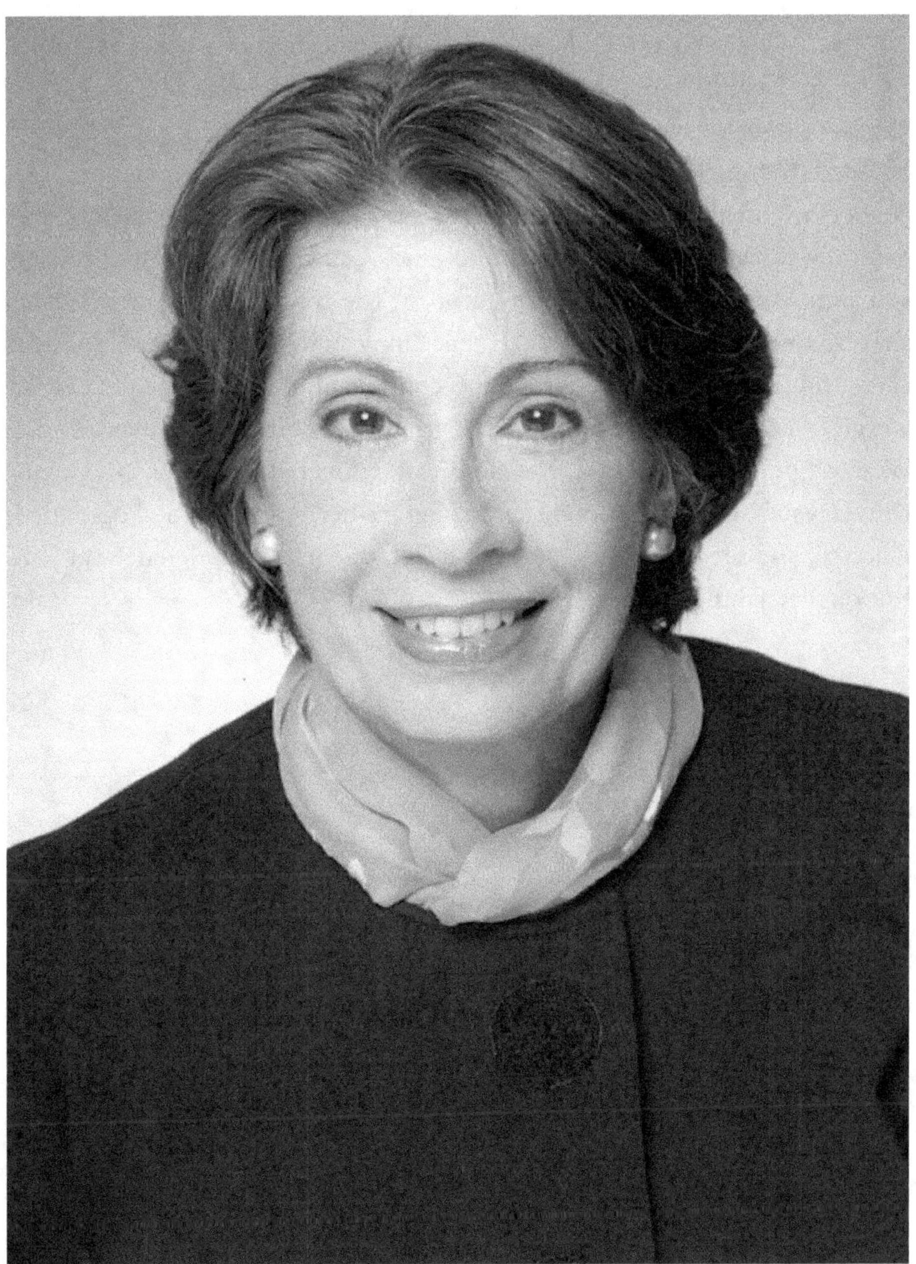

Dr. Beverly Winikoff, President, Gynuity Health Projects and Professor of Clinical Population and Family Health, Colombia Mailman School of Public Health

Dr. Beverly Winikoff, M.D., M.P.H., is the visionary behind Gynuity Health Projects, a global research NGO dedicated to advancing innovative approaches for enhancing women's reproductive health. With a rich background at the Population Council spanning 25 years where she served as Program Director for Reproductive Health and Senior Medical Associate, Dr. Winikoff has been at the forefront of pivotal research. As the principal investigator for the U.S. trials of mifepristone, she also directed studies in India, Cuba, China, and Vietnam. Her impactful career focuses on reproductive choice, contraception, abortion, and overall women's health. A magna cum laude graduate of Harvard University, Dr. Winikoff holds an M.D. from the New York University and an M.P.H. from the Harvard School of Public Health. Before her tenure at the Population Council, she served as the Assistant Director for Health Sciences at The Rockefeller Foundation.

Summary of the Podcast

In this podcast of Public Health Uncoded, Dr. Saroj Pachauri invited Dr. Beverely Winikoff a reproductive health specialist. Dr. Winikoff discussed the topic of abortion, focusing on its legalization in India and the variations in access and regulations across different countries. In her conversation with Dr. Pachauri, she mentioned that access to abortion services is influenced by both the medical system and legal/political factors. While some places allow midwives or nurses to provide surgical abortion services, others restrict it to doctors.

Highlighting the use of abortion pills, she mentioned that the technology has been available since the 1980s and has had a high success rate in the first trimester (7). She also spoke about the power and autonomy of women in making their own reproductive choices and the potential for ordering abortion pills online. She mentioned that the availability and accessibility of abortion-related drugs vary depending on the country and jurisdiction, with complexities arising from legal, scientific, and political factors (8). She and Dr. Pachauri discussed the ongoing debates and news surrounding abortion in the USA and the emergence of online platforms for purchasing abortion-related drugs. She provided an overview of abortion access, technology, and related issues in different parts of the world.

Scan the QR Code or follow the link to listen
https://thepopmovement.org/podcast-public-health-uncoded/

What is safe abortion?

W**hat is safe abortion?**

Safe abortion refers to the termination of a pregnancy through methods recommended by the World Health Organization (WHO) that are carried out by trained healthcare professionals in hygienic conditions. Safe abortion practices are critical for ensuring the health and wellbeing of women. Key aspects of safe abortion include:

1. **Medical Abortion**: The use of medications, such as mifepristone and misoprostol, to terminate a pregnancy. This method is effective and can be safely managed in various settings, including at home with proper guidance.
2. **Surgical Abortion**: Procedures such as vacuum aspiration and dilation and curettage (D&C) performed by trained healthcare providers in a clinical setting. These procedures are safe when performed under sterile conditions.
3. **Access to Care**: Ensuring that women have access to safe abortion services without barriers such as legal restrictions, lack of information, or financial constraints. This includes post-abortion care to manage any complications and provide contraceptive counseling.
4. **Training and Guidelines**: Health professionals should be adequately trained, and facilities should follow WHO guidelines to ensure the safety and efficacy of abortion procedures.
5. **Informed Consent and Counseling**: Women should receive compre-

hensive information about their options, the procedures, potential risks, and post-abortion care to make informed decisions.

References

World Health Organization (WHO):

WHO provides detailed guidelines and recommendations on safe abortion practices, emphasizing the importance of access to safe and legal abortion services to protect women's health. For more details, visit WHO's Safe Abortion Guidelines.

Guttmacher Institute:

The Guttmacher Institute conducts research and policy analysis on abortion, providing data and insights into the safety and accessibility of abortion services worldwide. Explore their resources at Guttmacher Institute's Abortion Page.

United Nations Population Fund (UNFPA):

UNFPA advocates for women's reproductive rights and access to safe abortion services as part of comprehensive sexual and reproductive health care. For more information, check UNFPA's Safe Abortion Page.

Centers for Disease Control and Prevention (CDC):

The CDC provides information on the safety and regulation of abortion procedures in the United States, including data on abortion-related complications and guidelines for healthcare providers. Visit CDC's Abortion Page.

International Planned Parenthood Federation (IPPF):

IPPF works globally to ensure access to safe and legal abortion services as part of comprehensive sexual and reproductive health care. They offer resources and advocacy tools on safe abortion. Visit IPPF's Safe Abortion Resources.

Ensuring access to safe abortion services is crucial for protecting women's health and upholding their reproductive rights.

PODCAST 4: HIV & AIDS

The recent surge of HIV infections is a serious cause of concern. There is a need to implement prevention and treatment measures to effectively control the spread of the infection.

The recent UNAIDS report states that HIV is in danger. HIV & AIDS programs are currently at risk due to the decrease in the response rate because of the COVID-19 pandemic. In 2022, one million more infections were reported than expected. Despite this alarming trend, only a fraction of the funds needed are available to address the demand for testing and treatment. The shortage of resources has created a gap of 20-30 percent globally. The goal to end the HIV/AIDS epidemic by 2030 appears to be elusive. The requirement is 30 billion dollars, but only 20-21 billion dollars are available. A significant number of new cases have been seen in young people, indicating a need to target services to specific population groups.

Communication strategies also need to be reassessed because the media landscape has changed over time. Young people are less interested in TV and radio campaigns and more engaged with social media platforms.

While treatment regimens have improved, adverse effects and long treatment still deter individuals from taking treatment. The supply chain also remains a weakness.

An approach that balances prevention and treatment is needed. In recent years, prevention has been neglected. It is important to revitalize old prevention methods, such as the condom, and implement newer, proven technologies, such as pre-exposure prophylaxis (PrEP). Governments should reduce the cost of PrEP to make it more affordable.

Communication campaigns addressing HIV prevention should be targeted to young people and adolescents and to key populations to inform them about HIV risks.

There is a need to increase political will, undertake advocacy, and mobilize resources to fill the funding gaps. Effective strategies should be implemented in collaboration with governments, advocates, and HIV/AIDS organizations worldwide.

The audience for this podcast discussion includes public health experts, research scientists, communication experts, policy planners, service providers, and users of services, especially young people and key populations.

Questions addressed

1. Why is the HIV/AIDS response in danger?
2. Where do we stand on treatment and how big is the gap?
3. How do we keep negative people negative?
4. Do we have adequate resources to reach the 95-95-95 targets?

Keywords

HIV/AIDS, HIV testing, key populations, UNAIDS, communication campaigns, and HIV prevention and treatment

Rajiv Dua

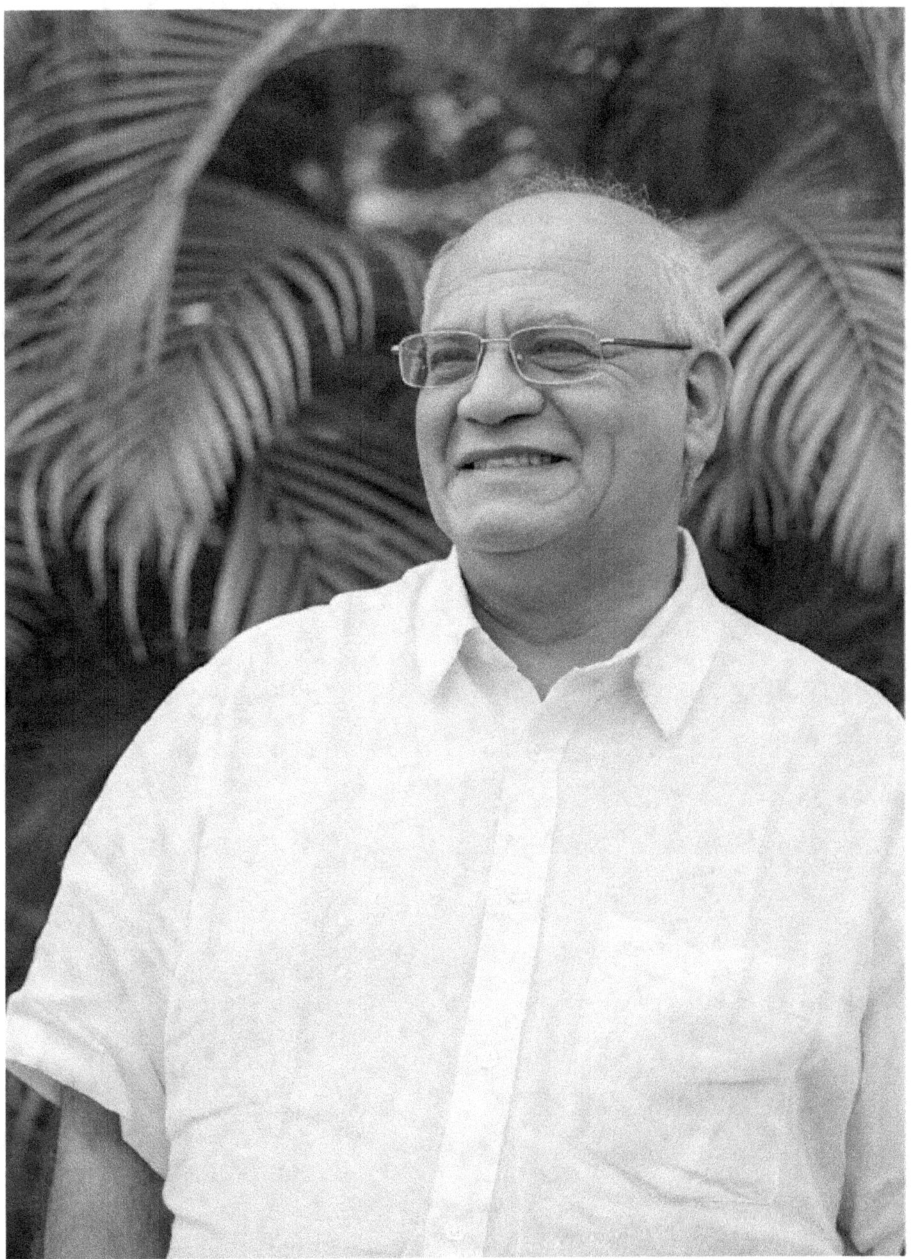

Rajiv Dua, Chief Executive, India HIV/AIDS Alliance

Rajiv Dua, a seasoned professional with over 33 years of experience in the health sector, has dedicated his career to improving health outcomes in various countries such as Bangladesh, India, Liberia, Nepal, the Philippines, and South Africa. In addition to his work in these countries, he has provided consultancy services in over 11 other countries. Mr. Dua's areas of expertise revolve around community health, marginalized populations, self-care, social marketing, developing cost-effective interventions, and risk management within the health sector. He has keen interest in the ethical use of Artificial Intelligence (AI) in healthcare and actively follows developments in this field.

Summary of the podcast

In this podcast of Public Health Uncoded, Dr. Saroj Pachauri and our special guest Mr. Rajiv Dua, an HIV/AIDS specialist, delved into the topic of the current status of HIV/AIDS in India and globally.

The recent UNAIDS report has highlighted that HIV is in danger (9). HIV/AIDS is currently at risk due to a decrease in response rates both prior to and following the COVID-19 pandemic. Mr. Dua talked about the issues that the report brought out. The report highlights that in 2022, one million more infections were reported than anticipated. Despite this alarming trend, only a fraction of the funds required were available to address the demand for testing, treatment, and medicines. Approximately 20-21 billion dollars were available. But the actual requirement is 30 billion dollars. Another concerning issue is that the global average for individuals who should be aware of their HIV status is 95 percent, leaving a 20 percent deficit. Thus, the challenge lies in improving this figure. A significant number of new infections have been observed among young people, indicating the need to shift campaign strategies to target specific groups since the existing approaches have proven to be ineffective. A reassessment of communication campaigns is imperative.

Talking about the challenges, Mr. Dua highlighted the proportion of HIV-positive individuals who are aware of their status and have access to treatment. He discussed the obstacles to increasing awareness. The media landscape has changed over time with traditional communication campaigns such as TV and radio spots being less effective among the current generation that is more engaged with social media platforms like Facebook and Instagram. Mr. Dua mentioned that treatment literacy was also a challenge. Although treatment regimens have improved, adverse effects and treatment fatigue still deter individuals from adhering to long-term treatment. He mentioned that supply chains for antiretroviral drugs also remain a weakness in the HIV/AIDS response. He discussed the strategies that could be adopted to reach out to more people with revised campaigns.

Mr. Dua emphasized the need for an approach that balances treatment and prevention. The shortage of resources was highlighted. There is an annual shortfall of approximately $10 billion. He mentioned that the current focus was on redirecting available resources to treatment programs as suppressing viral load reduces the chances of transmission. He stressed that both treatment and prevention should work together rather than being pitted against each other. He suggested revisiting and revitalizing old prevention methods such as condoms and implementing newer prevention technologies such as pre-exposure prophylaxis (PrEP). He proposed that governments should reduce the price of PrEP through negotiations with pharmaceutical industries. His major focus was on prevention. Mr. Dua suggested that HIV/AIDS prevention should be addressed through communication campaigns, particularly to reach and educate the younger populations, including adolescents and key populations, about the risks of HIV/AIDS.

Mr. Dua stated that there was a six percent decrease in the resources allocated to combating HIV/AIDS over the past two to three years despite an increase in the number of people affected by the disease. The required funding for HIV/AIDS programs was approximately $29 billion per year, while the currently available funds amounted to only $21 to $22 billion annually. This shortage of resources created a gap of around 25 to 30 percent globally, impeding efforts to end the epidemic by 2030, as promised. International donors had not kept pace with the growing need, resulting in a lack of political commitment and reduced funding.

He emphasized the need for increased political will, advocacy, and mobilization of resources to bridge the funding gap. Implementation of effective strategies and collaboration of governments, advocates, and HIV/AIDS organizations worldwide are necessary to adequately resource the response to the epidemic. Failure to address this issue could result in a resurgence of infections, especially among vulnerable populations.

Scan the QR Code or follow the link to listen
https://thepopmovement.org/podcast-public-health-uncoded/

What are HIV and AIDS?

What are HIV and AIDS?

HIV (Human Immunodeficiency Virus) is a virus that attacks the body's immune system, specifically the CD4 cells (T cells), which are crucial for immune defense. Over time, HIV can destroy so many of these cells that the body can't fight off infections and diseases. Without treatment, HIV can lead to the disease known as AIDS (Acquired Immunodeficiency Syndrome).

Key Points about HIV

Transmission: HIV is transmitted through contact with certain body fluids such as blood, semen, vaginal fluids, rectal fluids, and breast milk from a person who has HIV. It is commonly spread through unprotected sexual contact, sharing needles, or from mother to child during childbirth or breastfeeding.

Stages of HIV:

- **Acute HIV Infection**: This is the initial stage following exposure, where individuals may experience flu-like symptoms as the body responds to the virus.
- **Chronic HIV Infection**: Also known as the latent or asymptomatic stage, this period can last for several years, during which the virus

continues to replicate at low levels.

- **AIDS**: This is the most severe phase of HIV infection, characterized by a significantly weakened immune system, leading to opportunistic infections and certain cancers.

Diagnosis and Treatment:

- **Diagnosis**: HIV is diagnosed through blood tests that detect the presence of the virus or antibodies produced in response to the infection.
- **Treatment**: There is no cure for HIV, but it can be controlled with antiretroviral therapy (ART). ART helps reduce the viral load to undetectable levels, improving quality of life and reducing the risk of transmission.

Key Points about AIDS

1. **Definition**: AIDS is the final stage of HIV infection, marked by a severely damaged immune system. This is diagnosed when the number of CD4 cells falls below a critical level or when certain opportunistic infections or cancers develop.
2. **Symptoms**: Symptoms of AIDS can include rapid weight loss, recurring fever, extreme fatigue, prolonged swelling of lymph glands, and severe infections or diseases like tuberculosis, pneumonia, and certain cancers.
3. **Management**: While AIDS is life-threatening, early diagnosis and effective ART can prevent progression to this stage.

References

World Health Organization (WHO):

WHO provides comprehensive information on HIV and AIDS, including prevention, treatment, and global statistics. For more details, visit WHO's HIV/AIDS Page.

Centers for Disease Control and Prevention (CDC):

The CDC offers extensive resources on HIV/AIDS, including transmission, prevention, testing, and treatment guidelines. Visit CDC's HIV/AIDS Page.

UNAIDS:

UNAIDS leads the global effort to end AIDS as a public health threat. They provide detailed reports and data on the global HIV/AIDS epidemic. Explore their resources at UNAIDS.

National Institutes of Health (NIH):

The NIH's National Institute of Allergy and Infectious Diseases (NIAID) conducts research on HIV/AIDS and provides up-to-date information on treatment and prevention. Visit NIH's HIV/AIDS Page.

Mayo Clinic:

The Mayo Clinic offers comprehensive information on the symptoms, diagnosis, and treatment of HIV and AIDS. Check their resources at Mayo Clinic's HIV/AIDS Page.

Understanding HIV and AIDS is crucial for prevention, early diagnosis, and effective management, which can significantly improve the quality of life for those affected.

PODCAST 5: GENDER

Gender is a cross-cutting issue. It weaves through all sexual and reproductive issues. Gender disparities are prevalent worldwide but play out differently in various countries. The cost of ignoring gender concerns is high monetarily and socially. Gender problems are deeply entrenched in society and within the health system. These tenacious problems are difficult to overcome. Progress in improving gender equality has been disappointing in both developed and developing countries.

It is important to address the challenge of involving men and the need for educating them on sexual and reproductive health issues, understanding the set-back to gender equality caused by the COVID-19 pandemic, and examining the contradictions seen in some developing countries that have made progress in gender equality despite their poor socio-economic indicators.

The audience for this podcast discussion includes women advocates, researchers, policy planners, service providers, and users of services, especially women.

Questions addressed

1. How does gender disparity play out differently in developed and developing countries?
2. Why is gender-based violence a serious outcome of gender disparity?

3. What should be the priority strategies for achieving the SDG goal 5 given that we have regressed in achieving this goal due to COVD 19?
4. What are the costs of ignoring gender disparity?

Keywords

Gender disparity, COVID-19 pandemic, sustainable development goal 5 (SDG 5), male involvement, and developing nations

Madhu Bala Nath

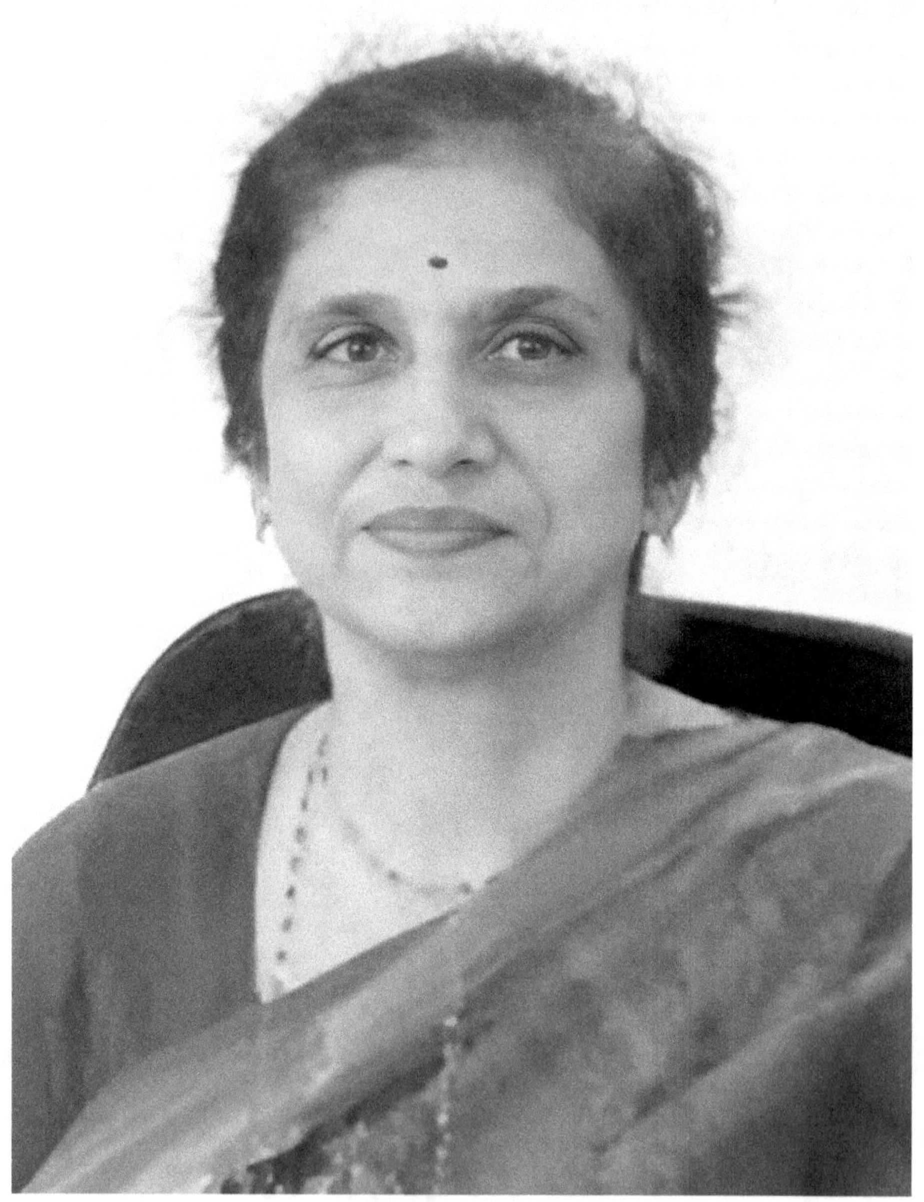

Madhu Bala Nath, Gender Specialist

Madhu Bala Nath, a gender specialist, has worked on issues related to gender, diversity, and inclusion across the developing sectors. She has worked with the Swedish International Development Authority (SIDA), the United Nations, the International Planned Parenthood Federation (IPPF), and Engender Health, New Delhi, India.

Summary of the podcast

In the two podcasts of Public Health Uncoded, Dr. Saroj Pachauri and our special guest, Ms. Madhu Bala Nath, discussed the topic of gender disparity.

The discussion began by highlighting the surprising fact that developing nations like Rwanda and Namibia rank among the top 10 countries in terms of gender equality. Ms. Nath provided a comprehensive report card of the progress made in addressing gender disparity from the 1980s until today.

She focused on the involvement of men in addressing gender disparity and the impact of the COVID-19 pandemic on achieving the targets of Sustainable Development Goal 5. Ms. Nath and Dr. Pachauri explored the challenges faced and discussed the need to provide male peers with education on sexual and reproductive health. They also discussed the need to understand the male perspective and the setbacks caused by the pandemic, which had affected women in terms of nutrition, health, and economics. Strategies to mitigate the impact of COVID-19 were examined as the pandemic played a significant role in hindering progress toward achieving SDG 5 (10).

Ms. Nath referred to the statistics cited in her chapter, "Cost of Ignoring Gender," in the book "Transforming Unequal Gender Relations: An Intersectional Perspective on Challenges and Opportunities." This book is edited by Dr. Saroj Pachauri and Dr. Ravi Verma (11).

Scan the QR Code or follow the link to listen
https://thepopmovement.org/podcast-public-health-uncoded/

If you find this book helpful, we would appreciate it if you left us a favorable review!

What is gender?

W**hat is gender?**

Gender refers to the roles, behaviors, activities, expectations, and societal norms that cultures and societies consider appropriate for men, women, and other gender identities. It is a complex concept that encompasses a range of identities and expressions beyond the binary notion of male and female. Key aspects of gender include:

1. **Gender Identity**: This is an individual's deeply felt internal experience of gender, which may be male, female, a blend of both, neither, or something else. It may or may not align with the sex assigned at birth.

2. **Gender Expression**: This refers to how an individual presents their gender to the world through behavior, clothing, hairstyles, voice, and other forms of presentation.

3. **Gender Roles**: These are the expectations and norms that societies and cultures have for individuals based on their perceived or assigned gender. These roles can vary widely across different societies and cultures and can change over time.

4. **Non-Binary and Gender Non-Conforming Identities**: These terms refer to gender identities that do not fit within the traditional binary of male and female. People who identify as non-binary may experience a gender that blends elements of both male and female, a gender that is neither, or a fluid gender.

5. **Gender Dysphoria**: Some individuals may experience discomfort or

distress due to a mismatch between their gender identity and the sex assigned at birth. Gender dysphoria is a recognized medical condition that can be alleviated through various forms of support, including social transition, hormone therapy, and surgery.

References

World Health Organization (WHO):

WHO provides information on gender and its impact on health, emphasizing the importance of gender equality and health equity. For more details, visit WHO's Gender Page.

American Psychological Association (APA):

APA offers resources and guidelines on understanding gender diversity and supporting individuals with diverse gender identities. Learn more at APA's Gender Page.

United Nations Development Programme (UNDP):

UNDP works towards gender equality and the empowerment of all women and girls. Their resources cover the social, economic, and political aspects of gender. Visit UNDP's Gender Equality Page.

National Center for Transgender Equality (NCTE):

NCTE provides resources and advocacy for transgender individuals, including information on gender identity and rights. Explore their resources at NCTE's Understanding Transgender Page.

Guttmacher Institute:

The Guttmacher Institute conducts research and provides insights on gender and reproductive health. Their publications offer valuable information on the intersection of gender and health. Visit Guttmacher Institute's Gender Page.

Understanding gender in all its diversity is crucial for fostering inclusion, equality, and respect for all individuals, regardless of their gender identity or expression.

PODCAST 6: HEALTH COMMUNICATION

Health communication is essential for delivering health information to the public. People require knowledge about health issues and where to access health services. This previously overlooked area is now acknowledged as crucial. It is not only important to disseminate information but also to gather feedback. Effective communication, a two-way process, is vital for enhancing public health.

It is important to understand the difference between information dissemination and health communication. Over time, health communication has evolved from traditional media to digital media. Too much information and miscommunication are challenges. Mis-communication posed a serious problem during the COVID pandemic. For example, there was large-scale miscommunication about vaccines. There is an urgent need for researchers and experts to play a more active role in sharing accurate information and countering misinformation, especially on social media. Health communication must promote appropriate actions and behaviors by encouraging dialogue and broad messaging.

This information would be of interest to communication experts, public health specialists, policy planners, and program implementors.

Questions addressed

1. What are the major communication challenges in the field of public health?
2. What was the impact of mis-communication on COVID-19 vaccination?
3. What do think about the misinformation on vaccine from the COVID-19 pandemic point of view?
4. What is the difference between information dissemination and health communication?

Keywords

Health communication, public health, medical communication, misinformation, internet explosion, behavior change, and vaccines

Anjali Nayyar

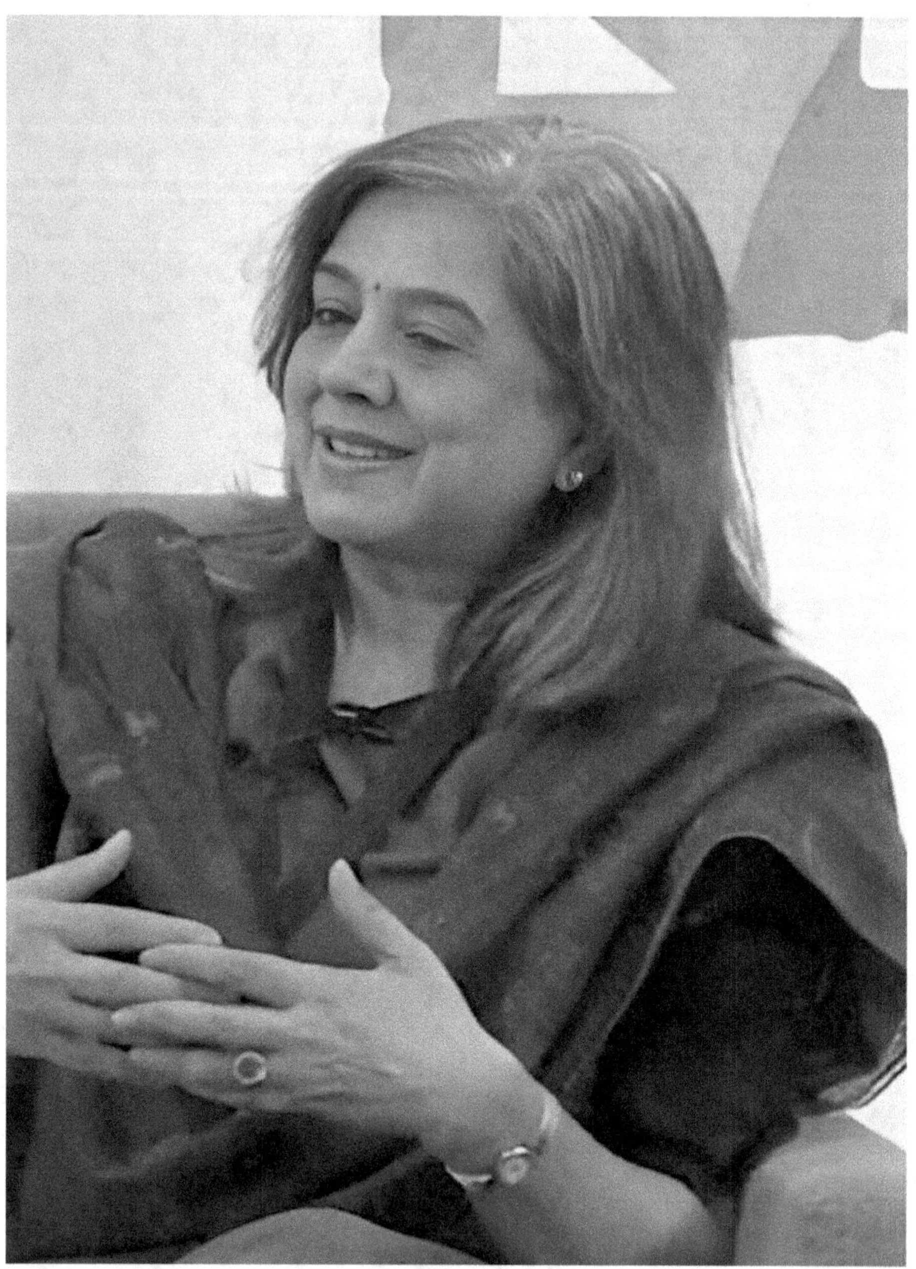

Anjali Nayyar, Executive Vice President, Global Health Strategies

Anjali Nayyar has more than 20 years of experience on global health issues. Her expertise lies in developing integrated programs, advocacy, and communications strategies aimed at impacting health policy and practice. She oversees the organization's programs in emerging markets in Asia and Africa working through four offices and independent consultants. Prior to joining Global Health Strategies (GHS), she served as Country Director for Program for Appropriate Technology on Health (PATH) in India. Preceding PATH, she worked with the International AIDS Vaccine Initiative (IAVI) for six years where she served initially as India Country Director and then as Vice President, Country and Regional Programs in New York. As Vice President, she led field operations and non-research and development programs in India, Brazil, South Africa, China, Kenya, Rwanda and Uganda. Ms. Nayyar also worked with the Population Council's Regional Office for South and East Asia as a Communications Specialist and Project Director. She is a member of the Confederation of Indian Industries' (CII's) National Committee on Public Health, the expert group on tuberculosis set up by a political forum called Global Coalition Against Tuberculosis, the *Pratigya* Campaign Advisory Group, and Uniting to Combat NTDs (National Tropical Diseases) Consultative Forum.

Summary of the podcast

In this podcast of Public Health Uncoded, Dr. Saroj Pachauri and our expert in health communications Ms. Anjali Nayyar, discussed the issue of health communication. They highlighted the differences between medical and public health communication noting that medical communications had historically received less attention while public health has emphasized strong communication programs. They discussed how the landscape of health communications had evolved over time with traditional media giving way to digital platforms like the internet and mobile phones.

Ms. Nayyar emphasizes the challenges of too much information and misinformation in health communications which was the case during the COVID-19 pandemic (12). She stressed the importance of experts and researchers playing a more prominent role in sharing accurate information and countering misinformation especially on social media. She also addressed the challenges of misinformation surrounding vaccines and emphasized the need for building confidence in vaccination.

The conversation concluded by providing a distinction between information dissemination and health communications highlighting that while dissemination was one-way targeted information, communications involved promoting actions and behaviors through dialogue and broader messaging. The critical role of communications in medical and public health contexts and the need to address challenges in disseminating accurate information and countering misinformation were discussed.

Scan the QR Code or follow the link to listen
https://thepopmovement.org/podcast-public-health-uncoded/

What is health communication?

What is health communication?

Health communication refers to promoting health information and education through various communication channels to enhance public health and wellbeing. It involves the strategic use of communication principles and methods to influence individuals, communities, and health professionals' attitudes, behaviors, and practices regarding health-related issues. Key components of health communications include:

1. **Information Dissemination**: Sharing accurate, timely, and accessible health information to the public through media campaigns, public service announcements, websites, social media, and other platforms.
2. **Behavior Change Communication (BCC)**: Strategies to influence and encourage positive health behaviors through targeted messages and interventions.
3. **Risk Communication**: Providing clear, accurate, and timely information about health risks to help individuals and communities make informed decisions during health crises, such as outbreaks or natural disasters.
4. **Health Literacy**: Enhancing individuals' ability to understand and use health information effectively to make informed health decisions.
5. **Interpersonal Communication**: Engaging in direct, one-on-one or group interactions between healthcare providers and patients to

improve health outcomes.

6. **Community Engagement**: Involving community members in planning and implementing health communication strategies to ensure cultural relevance and effectiveness.
7. **Feedback Mechanisms**: Collecting and using feedback from target audiences to improve the effectiveness of health communication efforts.

References

Centers for Disease Control and Prevention (CDC):

The CDC provides extensive resources and guidelines on health communication strategies, including best practices and case studies. For more details, visit CDC's Health Communication Page.

World Health Organization (WHO):

WHO offers a comprehensive overview of health communication, including its role in public health and guidelines for effective communication strategies. Explore more at WHO's Health Promotion Page.

National Institutes of Health (NIH):

The NIH's National Cancer Institute provides resources and tools for effective health communication, focusing on promoting health literacy and behavior change. Visit NIH's Health Communication Page.

U.S. Department of Health and Human Services (HHS):

HHS provides guidelines and resources on health communication and health literacy to support public health initiatives and improve health outcomes. Check HHS's Health Communication Page.

World Bank:

The World Bank offers resources on health communication, focusing on the impact of communication strategies on health outcomes in various regions. Visit World Bank's Health Communication Page.

Effective health communication is essential for promoting healthy behaviors, preventing diseases, and enhancing public health. It involves a multidisciplinary approach to ensure health information is accessible, accurate, and actionable.

PART 2: CHILD HEALTH

This section of the book will include two crucial discussions on child health.

Addressing the problem of child health is important, especially in developing countries where there are high rates of child mortality. Deaths of under-five-children are primarily due to communicable diseases and malnutrition. Immunization programs can significantly reduce child mortality. Malnutrition has traditionally taken the form of under-nutrition, resulting in stunting and wasting, which is an outcome of hunger. In recent years, obesity in young children has become a serious problem. While childhood obesity is increasing, it has been overlooked, especially in developing countries.

In recent years, we have witnessed the serious impacts of climate change on the health of children. This has resulted in high rates of respiratory diseases, including asthma and allergies, among children.

PODCAST 7: CHILDHOOD OBESITY

It is critical to understand the causes, consequences, and potential solutions for the problem of childhood obesity. While the problem of childhood obesity is increasing, it has been largely overlooked. Lifestyles, urban living, and eating habits affect childhood obesity. Lessons should be drawn from successful global practices. There is a need to design program strategies to scale up innovations. There are critical linkages between childhood obesity and non-communicable diseases (NCDs) like diabetes and cardiovascular diseases. Leveraging mobile technologies to engage and educate children, families, and communities is important. This could be a powerful intervention for bringing about behavioral change. There is a need for inter-sectoral collaboration and policy change to address the problem of childhood obesity.

This information would be of interest to nutritionists, medical experts, policy-planners, and researchers.

Questions addressed

1. What are the main causes of the rise in childhood obesity in recent years?
2. Is childhood obesity an urban problem, or is it prevalent in rural areas as well?
3. Among Asian Indian children, are body fat and abdominal adiposity contributing factors?

4. What are some of the global best practices to combat obesity that other countries can learn from?
5. What steps can be taken at the policy level to ensure that this problem does not go out of hand?

Keywords

Childhood obesity, malnutrition, nutritional challenges, developing countries, obesity prevention, and health interventions

Seema Chandra

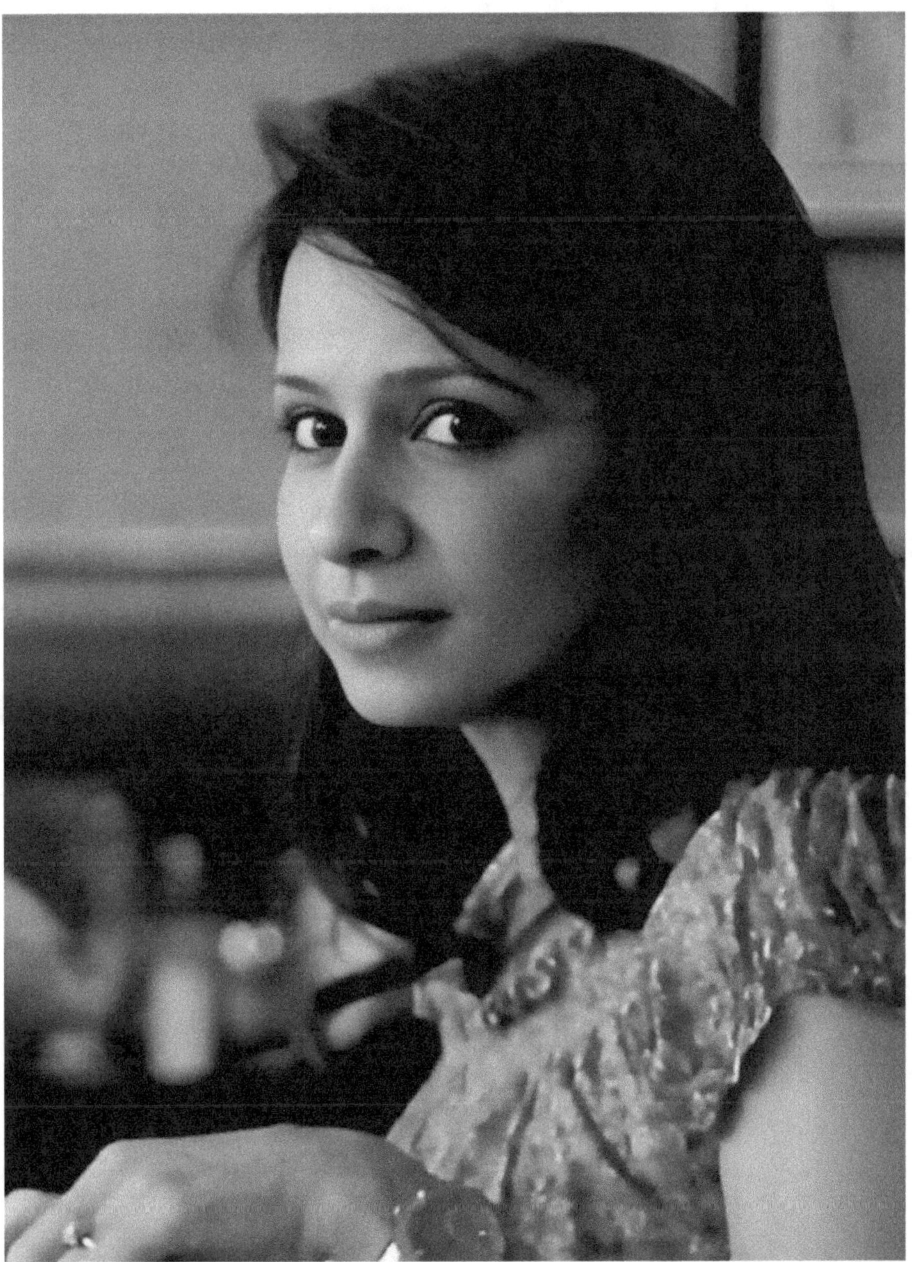

Seema Chandra, Creative Director at Editorji

Seema Chandra has had a career spanning the media and the wellness sectors. Her diverse roles include serving as the Creative Director at Editorji, an AI-based news and information app that delivers daily content on lifestyle, global health, nutrition, environment, and technology. She held the position of Managing Director at Smartcooky, an e-commerce venture focusing on health food and wellness products. Prior to that, she played a crucial role as the Food Editor in conceptualizing India's pioneering nutrition and health food show, "Good Food" aired on NDTV 24*7. She also contributed significantly to the launch of NDTV Good Times, India's first-ever lifestyle channel.

Ms. Chandra's academic dedication is evident in her achievements. In 2021, she obtained a master's in public health from New York University. She pursued courses at the University of California, Berkeley, concentrating on microeconomics, political economy, rhetoric, and organizational behavior. Her undergraduate studies earned her a bachelor of arts with honors in economics from Delhi University, where she specialized in public finance, economic systems, and economic history.

Summary of the podcast

In this podcast of Public Health Uncoded, Dr. Saroj Pachauri and Ms. Seema Chandra discussed childhood obesity, which is a growing and serious issue in developing countries. Ms. Chandra brought in her expertise in nutrition and communications to shed light on the causes, consequences, and potential solutions for this problem. She delved into various aspects of childhood obesity including it's prevalence, causes, urban and rural dynamics, economic factors, genetic influences, and health risks.

Ms. Chandra highlighted the alarming statistics on childhood obesity globally and in India and emphasized the need for urgent attention to problem. She explained that while efforts have been made to address under-nutrition, childhood obesity has been largely overlooked. She discussed how changes in living conditions, urbanization, dietary habits, and lifestyle factors have contributed to the rise of childhood obesity. Genetic factors and maternal obesity during pregnancy are also potential contributors.

Ms. Seema Chandra described successful global practices to combat childhood obesity. She cited examples from countries like Sri Lanka, Chile, and Bhutan that have implemented food-based dietary guidelines, labeling regulations, and school-based interventions. She emphasized the importance of scaling up innovative interventions by using digital technologies and developing behavior change strategies. She also discussed the connection between childhood obesity and non-communicable diseases (NCDs) like diabetes and cardiovascular diseases.

The conversation focused on the need for comprehensive research, evidence-based interventions, policy advocacy, and multi-sectoral collaboration to tackle the problem of childhood obesity effectively. Ms. Chandra suggested leveraging mobile technology, digital interventions, and creative methods to engage and educate children, families, and communities. She concluded optimistically by noting that concerted efforts could lead to meaningful progress in combating childhood obesity and it's associated health risks.

Scan the QR Code or follow the link to listen
https://thepopmovement.org/podcast-public-health-uncoded/

What is childhood obesity?

What is childhood obesity?

Childhood obesity is a serious medical condition affecting children and adolescents, characterized by excessive body fat that poses a health risk. It is determined using Body Mass Index (BMI) percentiles for age and sex. Childhood obesity is a major public health concern due to its association with various health problems and its potential to lead to obesity in adulthood.

Key Points about Childhood Obesity

Causes:

- **Diet**: High consumption of calorie-dense, nutrient-poor foods and beverages.
- **Physical Inactivity**: Sedentary lifestyle and lack of regular physical activity.
- **Genetics**: A family history of obesity can increase the likelihood.
- **Environmental Factors**: Lack of access to healthy foods, safe places to exercise, and education about healthy habits.
- **Psychological Factors**: Emotional stress and disorders can contribute to overeating and weight gain.

Health Consequences:

- **Physical Health**: Increased risk of type 2 diabetes, hypertension, high cholesterol, respiratory issues, and joint problems.
- **Mental Health**: Higher likelihood of experiencing low self-esteem, depression, and social isolation.
- **Long-term Risks**: A greater chance of becoming obese adults, which can lead to chronic health conditions such as heart disease, stroke, and certain cancers.

Prevention and Management:

- **Healthy Eating**: Encouraging balanced diets rich in fruits, vegetables, whole grains, and lean proteins while limiting sugary drinks and snacks.
- **Physical Activity**: Promoting at least 60 minutes of moderate to vigorous physical activity daily.
- **Behavioral Interventions**: Providing counseling and support to help children and families adopt healthier lifestyles.
- **Healthcare Guidance**: Regular monitoring and guidance from healthcare providers to track growth and provide tailored advice.

References

Centers for Disease Control and Prevention (CDC):

CDC provides comprehensive information on childhood obesity, including statistics, causes, consequences, and prevention strategies. For more details, visit CDC's Childhood Obesity Page.

World Health Organization (WHO):

WHO offers global perspectives on childhood obesity, addressing its prevalence, risk factors, and recommendations for prevention. Explore more at

WHO's Childhood Obesity Page.

Mayo Clinic:

Mayo Clinic provides detailed information on the causes, symptoms, and treatment of childhood obesity. Visit Mayo Clinic's Childhood Obesity Page.

National Institute of Diabetes and Digestive and Kidney Diseases (NIDDK):

NIDDK offers resources and research on childhood obesity, focusing on its impact on health and strategies for prevention and treatment. Learn more at NIDDK's Childhood Obesity Page.

American Academy of Pediatrics (AAP):

AAP provides guidelines and resources for healthcare professionals and parents to address and manage childhood obesity. Check AAP's Childhood Obesity Page.

Addressing childhood obesity requires a multifaceted approach involving parents, schools, healthcare providers, and communities to create supportive environments that promote healthy growth and development.

PODCAST 8: THE IMPACT OF CLIMATE CHANGE ON CHILD HEALTH

Climate change is a significant public health crisis. There are important connections between climate change and human health. Climate change significantly impacts children's health, increasing childhood morbidity. Climate change significantly impacts children's lives and the lives of caregivers and parents. There is an urgent need to assess the effects of asthma and allergies on the respiratory system in children. Climate change is a child rights crisis due to its disproportionate impact on children's health. There is an urgent need to educate parents and healthcare providers about this problem. There is also a need to strengthen public health systems to support children. It is important to empower youth about climate action.

The audience for this podcast includes climate scientists, public health experts, pediatricians, and policy planners.

Questions addressed

1. How does climate change impact children's health?
2. What are some equity considerations that should be taken into account when addressing climate change and child health?
3. What priority child health impacts should be addressed at the operational/programmatic and policy levels?

4. What key systems need to be strengthened to address the problem?
5. What is the role of children/youth in shaping climate resilience and mitigating problems?

Keywords

Climate change, children's health, mental health, air pollution, eco-anxiety, and climate education

Karina Weinstein

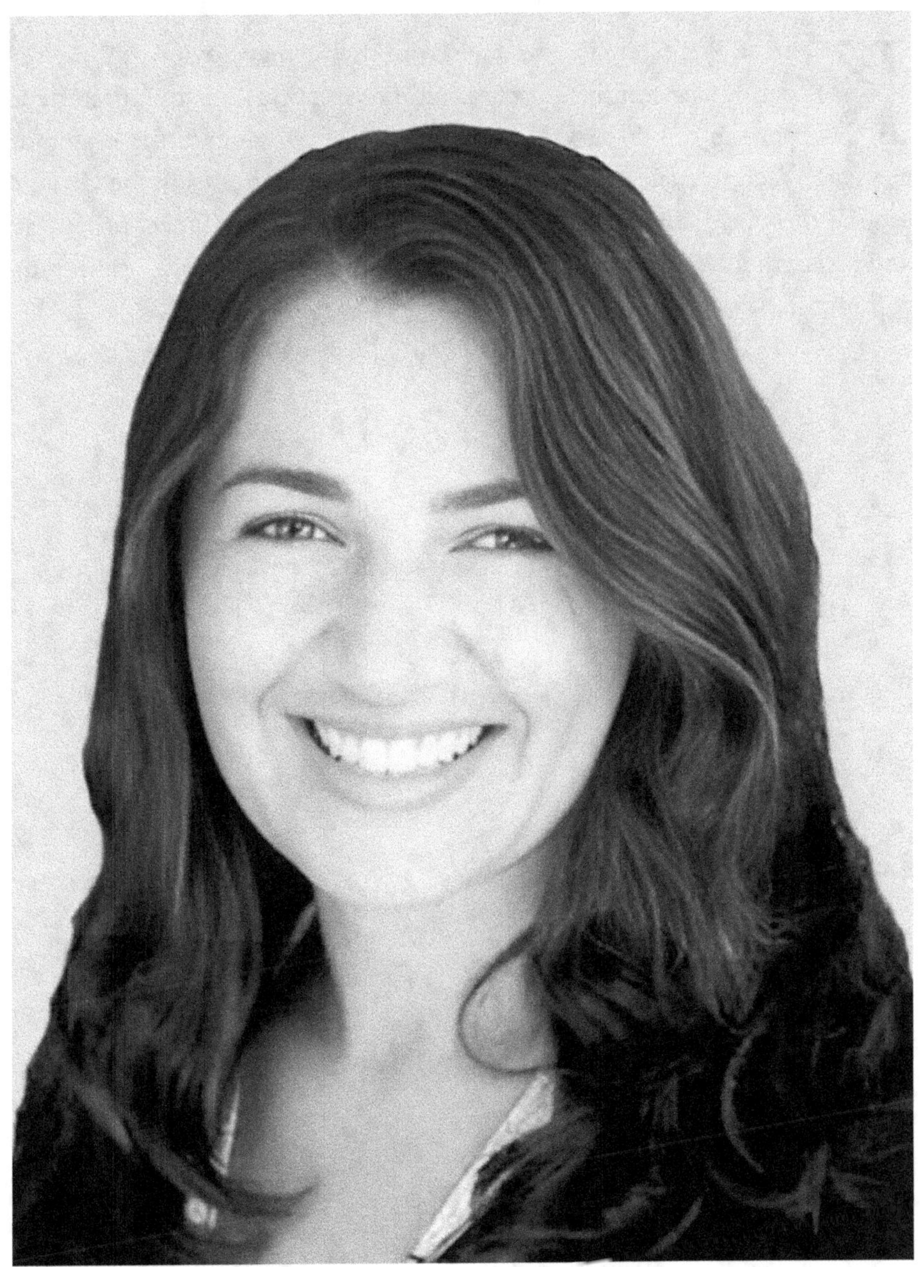

Karina Weinstein, Program Strategy and Innovation Director, FXB USA

Karina Weinstein is a refugee from the former Soviet Union who defied her immigrant community's expectations by pursuing a path in public service. Her work focuses on creating systemic change to facilitate access to opportunities for communities in the US and around the world. She has designed and developed social impact programs and strengthened grassroots organizations' capacity to serve immigrant communities.

Summary of the podcast

In this podcast of Public Health Uncoded, Dr. Saroj Pachauri invited Ms. Karina Weinstein, who discussed the significant impact of climate change on children's lives, caregivers, and surrounding systems like parents and schools, highlighting the importance of generating awareness of its tangible health effects such as asthma and allergies. Drawing from her personal experience, Ms. Weinstein advocated for translating research into public health action, portraying climate change as a child rights crisis due to it's disproportionate impacts on children's developing bodies (13). She highlighted the health impacts, especially mental health problems. She discussed the urgency for climate action to mitigate potential exacerbation of health issues. Prioritizing mental health, especially in children, she emphasized the need for comprehensive climate education and the importance of supporting parents and healthcare providers. Ms. Karina Weinstein stated that all sectors must recognize the link between climate change and health and incorporate this understanding within their programs. She stressed the importance of strengthening public health systems to support children facing climate change impacts. She highlighted a personal story from an activist in Bangladesh to underscore the importance of empowering youth to advocate for policy change. The discussion was based on individual examples that highlighted the importance of focusing on children's health in the context of climate change.

Scan the QR Code or follow the link to listen
https://thepopmovement.org/podcast-public-health-uncoded/

What are the impacts of climate change on child health?

What are the impacts of climate change on child health?

Climate change has a profound impact on child health, affecting both physical and mental wellbeing. Children are particularly vulnerable to the adverse effects of climate change due to their developing bodies and immune systems, dependency on caregivers, and specific physiological and psychological needs.

Key Impacts of Climate Change on Child Health

Increased Heat Exposure:

Heat Stress: Higher temperatures can lead to heat stress, dehydration, and heat-related illnesses in children.

Heat Waves: More frequent and severe heat waves pose significant risks, especially for infants and young children.

Air Quality Deterioration:

Respiratory Issues: Increased air pollution and allergens can exacerbate respiratory conditions such as asthma and bronchitis.

Long-term Effects: Chronic exposure to poor air quality can lead to long-term health problems, including reduced lung function and development.

Extreme Weather Events:

Natural Disasters: Hurricanes, floods, and wildfires can result in injuries, trauma, and displacement, disrupting children's lives and access to healthcare, education, and stable housing.

Mental Health: Exposure to natural disasters can lead to anxiety, depression, and post-traumatic stress disorder (PTSD) in children.

Food and Water Security:

Malnutrition: Climate change can affect food production and supply, leading to food insecurity and malnutrition, which are critical during childhood development.

Waterborne Diseases: Water availability and quality changes can increase the risk of waterborne diseases such as diarrhea, cholera, and other infections.

Vector-borne Diseases:

Increased Incidence: Warmer temperatures and changing precipitation patterns can expand the habitats of disease-carrying vectors like mosquitoes, leading to higher incidence of diseases such as malaria, dengue fever, and Zika virus.

Environmental Toxins:

Chemical Exposure: Climate change can exacerbate exposure to environmental toxins, such as heavy metals and pesticides, affecting children's growth and development.

References

World Health Organization (WHO):

WHO provides comprehensive information on the impact of climate change on health, including specific effects on children. For more details, visit WHO's Climate Change and Health Page.

Centers for Disease Control and Prevention (CDC):

The CDC offers resources and research on how climate change affects health, emphasizing the vulnerabilities of children. Learn more at CDC's Climate Change and Health Page.

United Nations Children's Fund (UNICEF):

UNICEF highlights the specific risks climate change poses to children and advocates for policies to protect children's health. Explore their resources at UNICEF's Climate Change Page.

American Academy of Pediatrics (AAP):

AAP provides guidelines and advocacy tools for addressing the impact of climate change on children's health. Visit AAP's Climate Change Page.

The Lancet Countdown on Health and Climate Change:

The Lancet Countdown provides annual reports on the health impacts of climate change, including data and analysis on how children are affected. Access their reports at The Lancet Countdown.

Addressing the impacts of climate change on child health requires coordinated efforts across sectors, including healthcare, policy, education, and community planning, to mitigate risks and enhance resilience.

PART 3: HEALTH IMPACTS OF CLIMATE CHANGE

This section of the book will feature six discussions on the critical and urgent topic of climate change and health. There is a growing concern about climate change's impacts on physical and mental health and wellbeing. Wide-ranging climate-related factors, including heat waves, air pollution, chemical pollution, and displacement of wildlife, impact human health. Research is urgently needed to study these factors and examine their impacts on human health. Research-based evidence should be used for designing programs and formulating policies, especially to prevent morbidity and mortality in children.

PODCAST 9: IMPACT OF CLIMATE CHANGE ON HUMAN HEALTH

Our planet is warming, and, consequently, it is having a serious impact on human health. There are far-reaching consequences of climate change on human health. Rising temperatures lead to more severe and more frequent weather events such as heat waves, floods, and droughts, which cause injuries, illnesses, and deaths. Warmer temperatures cause the spread of waterborne and vector-borne diseases. Droughts and extreme weather events disrupt food production and distribution systems and lead to malnutrition, particularly in vulnerable groups.

Air pollution caused by the burning of fossil fuels results in respiratory problems such as asthma. An uncertain future due to climate change is resulting in mental health problems. It is also causing increased anxiety, especially in children.

Unsustainable practices like deforestation and industrial agriculture are worsening the situation. The United Nations has called for a shift in eating habits, particularly reducing meat consumption, to decrease the environmental burden of livestock farming.

This information would be of interest to climate scientists, research scholars, and public health specialists.

Questions addressed

1. What health problems due to climate change are we already facing?
2. What is the second most disturbing effect of burning fossil fuels besides creating global warming?
3. How is our economic system increasing or even driving health risks created by the climate crisis?
4. How is growing food adding to health risks?

Keywords

Climate change, health problems, air pollution, mental health, fossil fuels, and food production

Antonio Sarmiento Galán

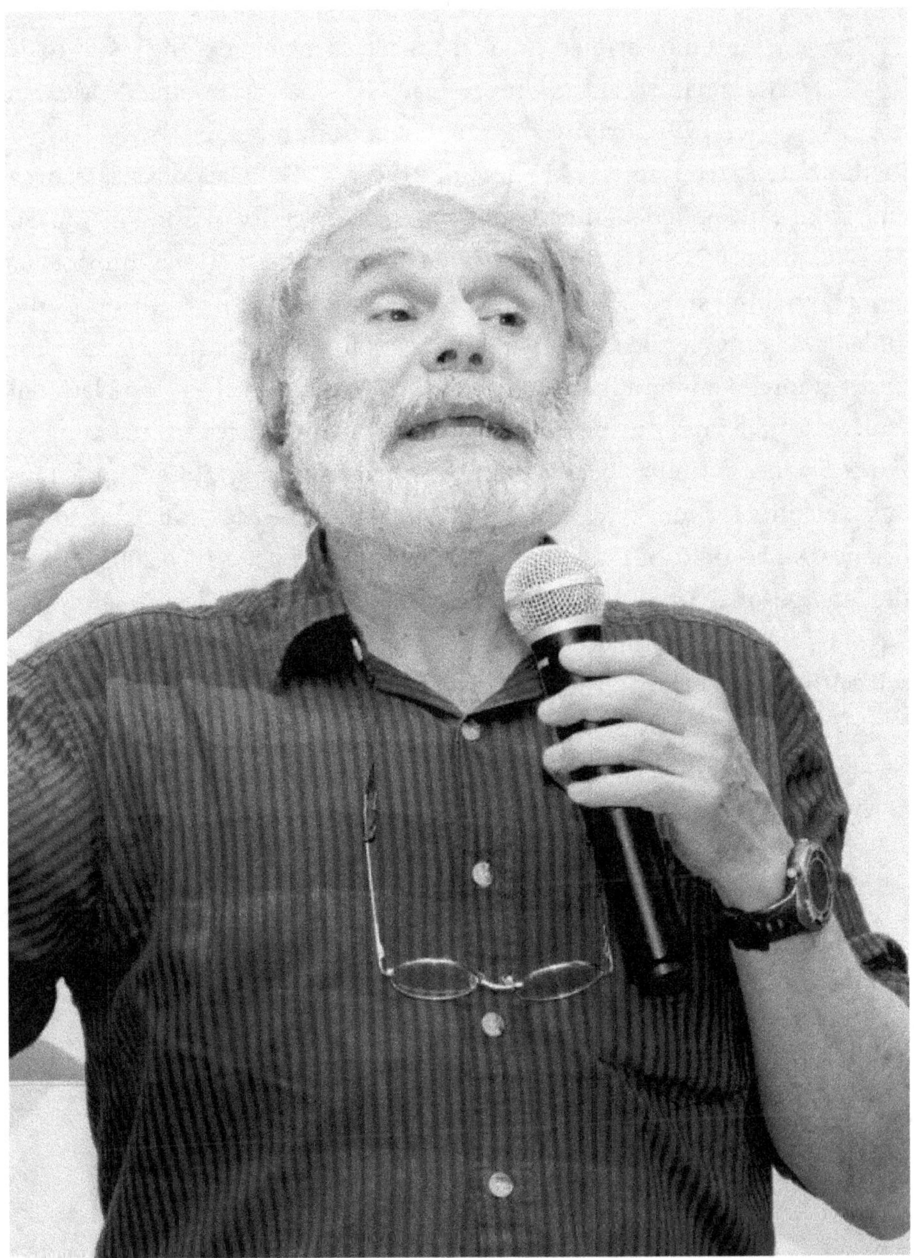

Dr. Antonio Sarmiento Galán, Scientist, Universidád Nacional Autónoma de México

Dr. Antonio Sarmiento Galán has been a member of the Instituto de Matemáticas at the Universidad Nacional Autónoma de México since 1999. Prior to his current appointment, he worked at the Instituto de Astronomía at México for 18 years. He has a physics degree and a Ph.D. in applied mathematics from the University of London (Queen Mary College, 1978-81). He has been examining the regional impacts of global warming since 2005. He offers a lecture course on anthropogenic global warming at the Universidad Nacional Autónoma de México for undergraduate and graduate students. In 1991, he received the National University Distinction for Young Academics in the area of Teaching in Exact Sciences. He has been a member of the Advisory State Council on Sustainability for the State of Morelos, México, of the Mexican Academy of Sciences since 1986, of the Morelos Academy of Sciences since 2003, and of the International Advisory Board of the Protect Our Planet Movement since 2016. His home is thermally auto-regulated and is free of fossil fuel use. It is self-sufficient in electric energy and water. More information available at: https://www.matcuer.unam.mx/~ansar/

Summary of the podcast

In this podcast of Public Health Uncoded Dr. Saroj Pachauri was joined by Dr. Antonio Galan, a leading climate scientist, to discuss the far-reaching consequences of climate change on human health.

Dr. Galan shared his insights on how various factors caused by a warming planet are affecting our wellbeing. The conversation covered:

- Increased dangers from extreme weather: Rising temperatures lead to more frequent and severe weather events like heat waves, floods, and droughts, causing injuries, illnesses, and deaths.
- Spread of waterborne and vector-borne diseases: Warmer temperatures and floods create ideal breeding grounds for mosquitoes and other insects, increasing the risk of diseases like malaria and dengue fever (14).
- Malnutrition threats: Droughts and extreme weather disrupt food production and distribution systems, leading to malnutrition, particularly in vulnerable communities.
- Respiratory problems on the rise: Air pollution caused by burning fossil fuels aggravates respiratory problems like asthma, posing a serious health risk.
- Mental health concerns: An uncertain future caused by climate change is leading to increased anxiety, especially among children.
- The role of fossil fuels: Burning fossil fuels is a major contributor to air pollution and greenhouse gas emissions, directly impacting human

health.

The discussion explored how unsustainable practices like deforestation and industrial agriculture worsen the situation. Dr. Galan mentioned the United Nation's call for a shift in eating habits, particularly reducing meat consumption, to lessen the environmental burden of livestock farming.

This podcast discussion provided a thought-provoking look at the far-reaching consequences of climate change on human health.

Scan the QR Code or follow the link to listen
https://thepopmovement.org/podcast-public-health-uncoded/

What are the impacts of climate change on human health?

What are the impacts of climate change on human health?

Key Impacts of Climate Change on Human Health

Increased Heat-Related Illnesses:

- **Heat Stress and Heat Stroke**: Rising temperatures and more frequent heatwaves lead to increased cases of heat stress and heat-related illnesses.
- **Cardiovascular and Respiratory Disorders**: Extreme heat can exacerbate cardiovascular and respiratory conditions, particularly among the elderly and those with pre-existing health conditions.

Poor Air Quality:

- **Respiratory Diseases**: Increased levels of air pollutants, such as ground-level ozone and particulate matter, worsen respiratory conditions like asthma and chronic obstructive pulmonary disease (COPD).
- **Allergies**: Higher temperatures and carbon dioxide levels can increase the concentration of allergens like pollen, leading to more severe allergy symptoms.

Changes in Vector-Borne Diseases:

- **Expanded Habitats**: Warmer temperatures and changing precipitation patterns expand the habitats of vectors such as mosquitoes and ticks, increasing the incidence of diseases like malaria, dengue fever, Zika virus, and Lyme disease.

Water and Food Security:

- **Waterborne Diseases**: Changes in precipitation patterns and increased temperatures can lead to water scarcity and contamination, increasing the risk of waterborne diseases such as cholera and dysentery.
- **Food Safety and Nutrition**: Climate change can disrupt food production, leading to malnutrition and foodborne illnesses due to the proliferation of pathogens in warmer conditions.

Mental Health Effects:

- **Stress and Anxiety**: The stress of dealing with extreme weather events, displacement, and the uncertainty of climate change impacts can lead to increased anxiety, depression, and other mental health issues.
- **Post-Traumatic Stress Disorder (PTSD)**: Survivors of natural disasters such as hurricanes, floods, and wildfires may experience PTSD and other long-term psychological effects.

Extreme Weather Events:

- **Injuries and Fatalities**: Natural disasters such as hurricanes, floods, and wildfires can cause direct physical harm, injuries, and fatalities.
- **Displacement and Homelessness**: Extreme weather events can lead to displacement, loss of homes, and disruption of communities, affecting overall wellbeing and access to healthcare.

Disruption of Healthcare Services:

- **Healthcare System Strain**: Increased demand for medical services during and after extreme weather events can strain healthcare systems, limiting access to care and resources.
- **Infrastructure Damage**: Damage to healthcare facilities and infrastructure can hinder delivering essential health services.

References

World Health Organization (WHO):

WHO provides extensive information on the health impacts of climate change, including reports and guidelines for addressing these challenges. For more details, visit WHO's Climate Change and Health Page.

Centers for Disease Control and Prevention (CDC):

The CDC offers resources and research on the health effects of climate change, emphasizing preparedness and adaptation strategies. Learn more at CDC's Climate and Health Page.

National Institutes of Health (NIH):

NIH provides research and information on the various ways climate change affects health, focusing on both direct and indirect impacts. Visit NIH's Climate Change and Health Page.

The Lancet Countdown on Health and Climate Change:

The Lancet Countdown publishes annual reports on the global health impacts of climate change, offering comprehensive data and analysis. Access their reports at The Lancet Countdown.

Environmental Protection Agency (EPA):

The EPA provides information on the health impacts of climate change in the United States, including detailed reports and resources for communities. Explore their resources at EPA's Climate Change and Human Health Page.

Addressing the health impacts of climate change requires coordinated efforts across healthcare, policy, education, and community planning to mitigate risks and enhance resilience.

PODCAST 10: SARGASSUM, A BROWN SEAWEED

The problem of sargassum is relatively new. This brown seaweed poses a serious threat to pristine beaches. This emerging multifarious problem affects more than 20 countries and has spread from the Caribbean Sea to the Atlantic Ocean. Research indicates that sargassum impacts human health and causes air pollution.

Sargassum affects human health and marine life. Heavy metals and toxins associated with sargassum impact the health of coastal communities. Research undertaken by the POP (Protect Our Planet) team to study its health impacts showed that sargassum affects the physical and mental health of the people exposed to it.

The audience for this podcast discussion includes climate scientists, research scholars, public health experts, and oceanographers.

Questions addressed

1. What is causing the problem of sargassum?
2. What is causing this massive movement of sargassum?
3. What are the effects of sargassum on human health and air pollution?

Keywords

Sargassum, climate change, health risks, Mexico, economic impact, Caribbean beaches, and environmental research

Norma Patricia Muñoz Sevilla

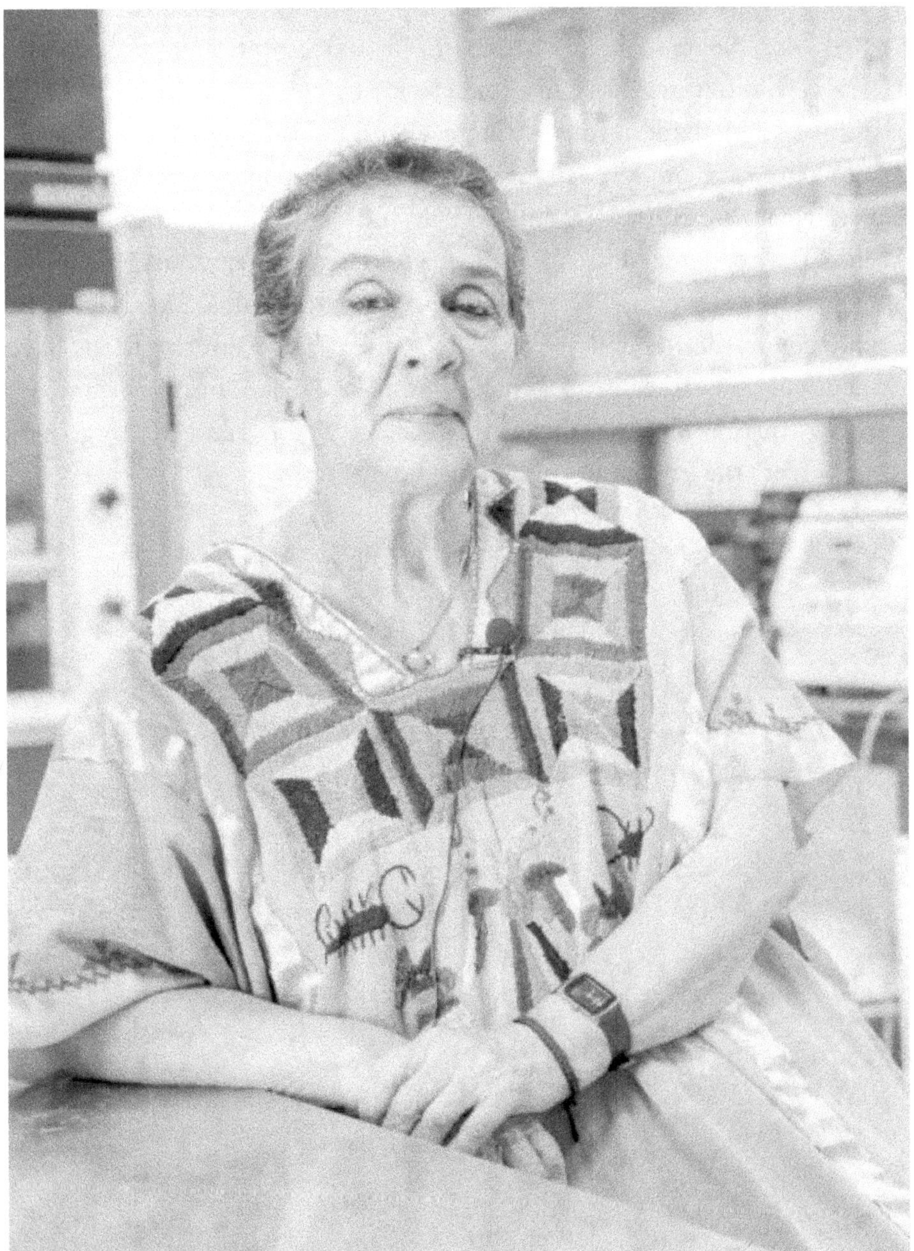

Dr. Norma Patricia Munoz, Honorary Mentor, POP (Protect Our Planet)
Movement and Researcher and Professor at Instituto Politecnico Nacional (IPN)

Dr. Norma Patricia Munoz holds a doctorate in oceanography biology and has had a remarkable career as an educator, having trained numerous masters and doctoral students. With 59 research projects and over 310 presentations to her name, she is a prominent figure in marine resource management and environmental impact. Dr. Muñoz is a recognized member of several environmental organizations. She currently serves as President of the Climate Change Council of the Presidency of the Republic of Mexico. Her extensive contributions have earned her numerous awards, including the "Great Woman of the 21st Century" distinction, the "Order of Academic Palms, and the Degree of Knight" from the French Republic.

Summary of the podcast

In this podcast of Public Health Uncoded, Dr. Saroj Pachauri and Dr. Norma Patricia Muñoz, a distinguished marine biologist, delved into the largely unknown issue of sargassum and its impact on health. (15). This emerging problem, widely unrecognized by the general public and the climate field, has been diligently researched by the POP (Protect Our Planet) Movement team, led by experts Dr. Pachauri and Dr. Munoz. This research sheds light on the multifaceted nature of sargassum, a threat spreading from the Caribbean Sea to the Atlantic Ocean and affecting more than 20 countries. Marine life is suffering, and the coastal communities are largely unaware of the impending impact of sargassum.

The research found that less than one percent of the population was aware of the heavy metals and toxins associated with sargassum. Further insights into sargassum and its connection to climate change can be found in the forthcoming book Climate and Health Nexus: Unraveling the Connections, edited by Dr. Saroj Pachauri and Dr. Ash Pachauri.

Scan the QR Code or follow the link to listen
https://thepopmovement.org/podcast-public-health-uncoded/

What is sargassum and how does it affect human health?

What is sargassum and how does it affect human health?

Sargassum is a genus of large brown seaweed (algae) that floats in island-like masses and is commonly found in the Sargasso Sea in the Atlantic Ocean. These seaweeds are notable for their buoyant properties, allowing them to form extensive mats on the ocean surface.

Impacts of Sargassum on Human Health

Respiratory Issues:

- **Hydrogen Sulfide Gas**: When sargassum decomposes, it releases hydrogen sulfide (H_2S), which can cause respiratory problems, especially in individuals with asthma or other respiratory conditions. Symptoms include eye irritation, coughing, shortness of breath, and headaches.

Skin Irritation:

- **Direct Contact**: Physical contact with sargassum or its decomposing matter can cause skin irritation and rashes. The seaweed may also harbor small marine organisms that can cause further irritation.

Water Quality:

- **Decomposition in Coastal Waters**: Large accumulations of sargassum can lead to oxygen depletion as it decomposes, creating hypoxic (low oxygen) conditions that can harm marine life and disrupt local ecosystems. This can indirectly affect human health by impacting local fisheries and food security.

Nuisance and Economic Impact:

- **Tourism and Fisheries**: Large sargassum blooms can accumulate on beaches, creating a foul odor and an unpleasant environment for tourists. This can negatively impact local economies reliant on tourism and fisheries, leading to economic stress that can have health consequences for affected communities.

References

World Health Organization (WHO):

WHO provides information on various environmental health issues, including the impacts of marine phenomena like sargassum on public health. For more details, visit WHO's Environmental Health Page.

Centers for Disease Control and Prevention (CDC):

The CDC offers guidelines and information on dealing with environmental health risks, including the potential health impacts of sargassum. Visit CDC's Environmental Health Page.

National Oceanic and Atmospheric Administration (NOAA):

NOAA provides comprehensive resources on sargassum, its environmental impacts, and how it affects human health. Explore more at NOAA's sargassum page.

United Nations Environment Program (UNEP):

UNEP addresses global environmental issues and reports on phenomena like sargassum's impact on ecosystems and human health. Visit UNEP's Marine Ecosystems Page.

Research Articles:

Medical Journal of Australia: A study detailing the health effects of hydrogen sulfide exposure from decomposing sargassum. Access the article here.

Marine Pollution Bulletin: An article on sargassum influxes' environmental and health impacts in the Caribbean. Find the article here.

Addressing the health impacts of sargassum requires coordinated efforts between environmental scientists, public health officials, and local communities to mitigate risks and manage affected areas effectively.

PODCAST 11: IMPACTS OF PERSISTENT ORGANIC POLLUTANTS AND ENDOCRINE DISRUPTING CHEMICALS ON HEALTH

Persistent organic pollutants (POPs) and endocrine disrupting chemicals (EDCs) are widespread and impact human health. These chemicals cause permanent damage at the fetal stage and can also cause cancer, reproductive diseases, and type 2 diabetes.

Europe and the USA have strict laws; they conduct regular research and monitor these chemicals. India's efforts have, however, have not been adequate. India is a member of global treaties such as the Stockholm Convention on POPs. India has made some efforts and is moving forward with the India Implementation Plan (16). It has also drafted a policy, but much more work is needed to tackle this problem. Limited research, inadequate resources, and non-compliance with existing policies exist. To effectively address this problem, the technical, administrative, and financial infrastructure must be improved urgently.

This podcast will interest climate scientists, public health professionals, research scholars, and policy-makers.

Questions addressed

1. What is being done to reduce chemical pollutants such as persistent organic pollutants (POPs) and endocrine disrupting chemicals (EDCs)?
2. What are the health impacts of these hazardous chemicals?
3. What are the learnings from research studies, and what is the general public's awareness of the health impacts of these hazardous chemicals?

Keywords

Endocrine disrupting chemicals (EDCs), persistent organic pollutants (POPs), chemical pollution, health impacts, Stockholm Convention, and chemical management and safety

Girija Bharat

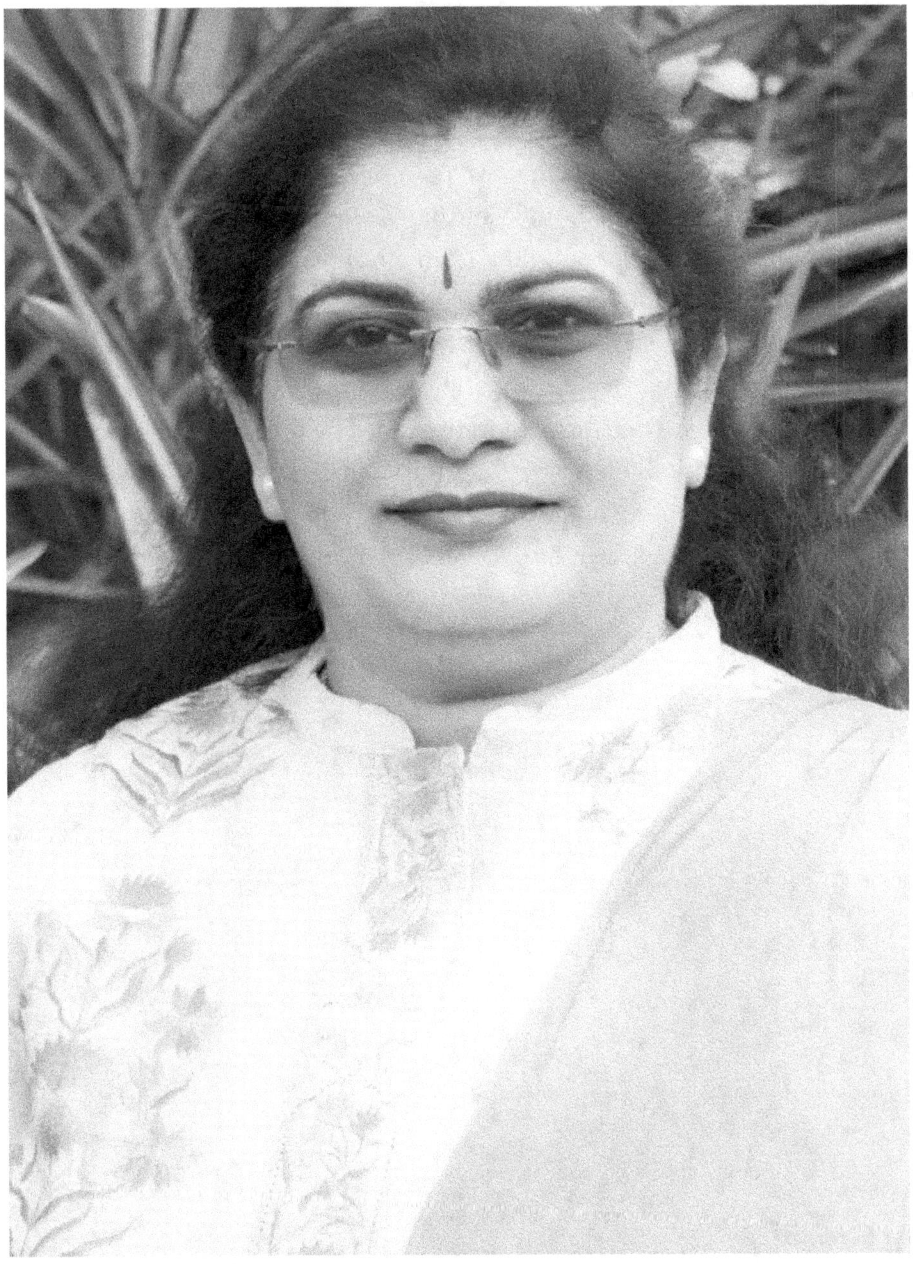

Dr. Girija Bharat, Managing Director, Mu Gamma Consultants

D r. Girija K Bharat, Managing Director, Mu Gamma Consultants, is a respected international expert with 30 years of experience in water quality. She specializes in water resource management, water supply and sanitation, chemical pollution control, and environmental management. She has a Ph.D. in chemistry from the Laxminarayan Institute of Technology (LIT), Nagpur. She is an alumna of esteemed institutions like the Indian Institute of Technology, Dhanbad and the George Mason University, USA. Dr. Bharat has published 128 research papers. Her contributions have earned her prestigious awards including the Glory of India 2021, Women Transforming India Award by the National Institute for Transforming India (NITI) Aayog 2021, the Global Environment Award 2020, the Save the Environment Award 2021, the Aqua Excellence Award 2020, and the Exceptional Women of Excellence Award of the Women Economic Forum in 2019.

Summary of the podcast

In this podcast of Public Health Uncoded, Dr. Saroj Pachauri and our expert, Dr. Girija Bharat, discussed endocrine-disrupting chemicals, their widespread presence, and their impact on human health.

During the conversation, Dr. Pachauri simplified the concept of endocrine-disrupting chemicals (EDCs) and discussed the different types of EDCs and persistent organic pollutants (POPs) (17)(18). She highlighted their properties, presence, and impact on various species in the ecosystem, including humans.

Dr. Bharat focused on the ubiquity of these chemicals and how they biomagnify, leading to health effects at different stages of life. She emphasized that the timing and level of exposure determined the nature and severity of their effects, including permanent damage during the fetal stage and effects on cancer, reproductive disorders, and type 2 diabetes in adulthood.

The conversation then shifted to what the world is doing about POPs and EDCs. Europe and America have strict laws and conduct regular research in this area to categorize chemicals based on their harmfulness. However, India's efforts are either not effectively communicated or are slow. Dr. Bharat explained India's approach, including its participation in global treaties such as the Stockholm Convention on POPs and the National Implementation Plan (NIP) for chemicals.

India is working on the NIP, which focuses on seven new chemicals. To replace the existing regulations, a draft policy called CMSR (Chemical Management and Safety Rules) is being developed. This policy resembles the European Union's REACH (Registration Evaluation Authorization and Restriction of Chemicals) framework.

Dr. Bharat mentioned that in spite of efforts made, there is still a lot to be done to manage chemicals safely. Existing gaps included a lack of credible data due to limited research, insufficient resources, and non-compliance with existing policies. There is a need to improve the technical, administrative, and financial infrastructure.

Scan the QR Code or follow the link to listen
https://thepopmovement.org/podcast-public-health-uncoded/

What are Persistent organic pollutants (POPs)?

What are Persistent organic pollutants (POPs)? What are their impacts and the impacts of endocrine disrupting chemicals (EDCs) on health?

Persistent organic pollutants (POPs) are toxic chemicals that adversely affect human health and the environment. They persist in the environment for long periods, bioaccumulate through the food web, and pose a risk of causing adverse effects. Examples include dioxins, polychlorinated biphenyls (PCBs), and pesticides like DDT.

Endocrine Disrupting Chemicals (EDCs) are substances that can interfere with organisms' hormonal systems. Many POPs are also classified as EDCs because they can mimic or interfere with the body's endocrine system, leading to various health issues.

Key Impacts on Health

Reproductive Health:

- **Fertility issues**: Exposure to EDCs can lead to reduced fertility in both men and women. Chemicals such as phthalates and bisphenol A (BPA) have been linked to lower sperm quality and decreased reproductive success.

- **Developmental effects**: In utero and early life exposure to EDCs can result in developmental abnormalities, such as genital malformations and altered timing of puberty.

Cancer:

- **Hormone-related cancers**: POPs and EDCs have been linked to an increased risk of hormone-related cancers, including breast, prostate, and testicular cancer. This is due to their ability to mimic or interfere with natural hormones in the body.

Neurological Effects:

- **Neurodevelopmental disorders**: Prenatal and early life exposure to certain POPs and EDCs has been associated with neurodevelopmental disorders, such as attention deficit hyperactivity disorder (ADHD) and autism spectrum disorders (ASD).

Immune System:

- **Immunotoxicity**: Some POPs can weaken the immune system, making individuals more susceptible to infections and diseases. For example, dioxins and PCBs have been shown to impair immune function.

Metabolic Disorders:

- **Obesity and diabetes**: EDCs have been linked to metabolic disorders, including obesity and type 2 diabetes. Chemicals like BPA and certain flame retardants can disrupt metabolic processes, increasing fat storage and insulin resistance.

How POPs create endocrine disrupting chemicals

1. **Chemical stability**: POPs are chemically stable and resistant to degradation, allowing them to persist in the environment for extended periods.
2. **Bioaccumulation and biomagnification**: POPs accumulate in the fatty tissues of organisms and biomagnify up the food chain, leading to higher concentrations in top predators, including humans.
3. **Molecular mimicry**: Many POPs can mimic natural hormones (e.g., estrogen and androgen) and bind to hormone receptors, disrupting normal hormonal functions.
4. **Interference with hormone production and metabolism**: POPs can interfere with the production, release, transport, metabolism, and elimination of natural hormones, disrupting the endocrine system.

References

World Health Organization (WHO):

WHO provides extensive information on the health effects of POPs and EDCs, including research and guidelines for reducing exposure. For more details, visit WHO's Endocrine Disruptors Page and WHO's POPs Page.

United States Environmental Protection Agency (EPA):

The EPA offers resources and research on POPs, including their sources, environmental persistence, and health impacts. Explore more at EPA's Persistent Organic Pollutants Page and EPA's Endocrine Disruptors Page.

National Institute of Environmental Health Sciences (NIEHS):

NIEHS provides information on the health effects of EDCs and POPs, emphasizing research findings and public health implications. Visit NIEHS's Endocrine Disruptors Page.

Stockholm Convention on Persistent Organic Pollutants:

An international treaty aimed at eliminating or restricting the production and use of POPs. The convention's website provides detailed information on the chemicals covered and efforts to mitigate their impacts. Access the resources at Stockholm Convention.

National Institutes of Health (NIH):

NIH offers research articles and resources on the impact of EDCs on human health, focusing on various health outcomes and mechanisms of action. Learn more at NIH's Endocrine Disruptors Page.

Understanding and mitigating the impacts of POPs and EDCs is crucial for protecting public health and ensuring a safer environment.

PODCAST 12: THE COVID-19 PANDEMIC

The COVID-19 pandemic has impacted every life in every country. No one has escaped from its effects. This pandemic has had health, social, economic, and political consequences. Since the infection spread from animals to humans, COVID-19 brought the problem of zoonotic diseases into focus.

It is important to undertake intersectoral programs and adopt a comprehensive, whole-government strategy. It is also important to leverage technology to foster collaboration between urban and rural areas, promote strong leadership, and encourage social participation. There is a need to remain vigilant.

This podcast discussion focused on India. It would interest public health specialists, researchers, policy planners, and service providers.

Questions addressed

1. COVID cases are still happening all over the world; is the worst over?
2. What role did vaccination play in combating the COVID-19 pandemic?
3. Have governments implemented fundamental changes in responding to public health crises like COVID? Are they better prepared to tackle future pandemics?

Keywords

Public health, COVID-19 pandemic, vaccination strategy, government response, healthcare infrastructure, and scientific collaboration

Bulbul Sood

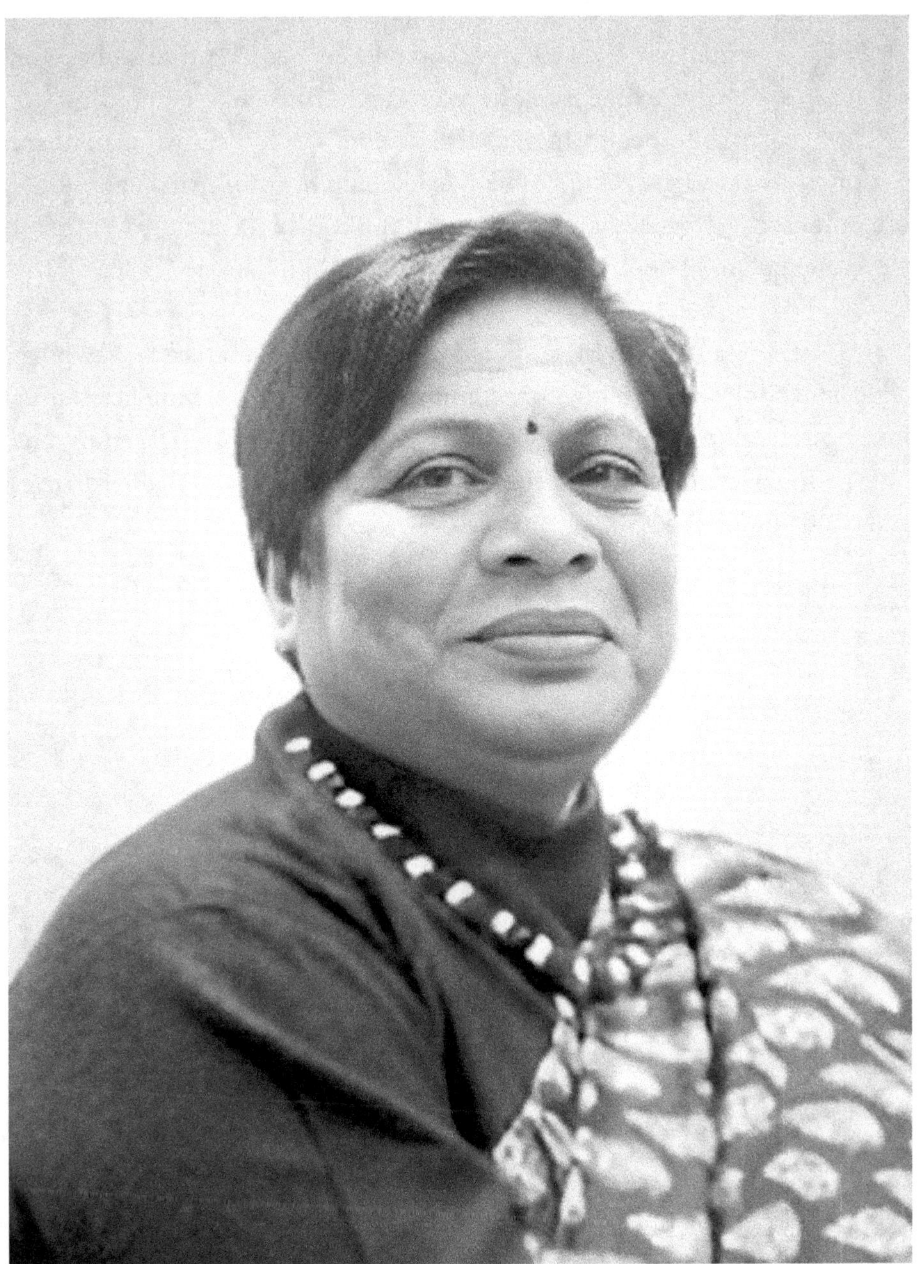

Dr. Bulbul Sood is an independent senior strategic advisor

Dr. Bulbul Sood is a highly accomplished medical professional with extensive expertise. She holds an MBBS degree and a master of public health (MPH). Dr. Sood serves as an independent senior strategic advisor and has held leadership positions throughout her career including former Country Director, Jhpiego-India and the Centre for Development and Population Activities (CEDPA), India.

Dr. Sood's areas of expertise include reproductive, maternal, newborn, child, and adolescent health, non-communicable diseases, women's cancer, infectious diseases (including COVID-19), health system strengthening, and international health. She is a prolific writer with over 40 published articles and contributions to book chapters.

Summary of the podcast

In this podcast of Public Health Uncoded, Dr. Saroj Pachauri and our special guest Dr. Bulbul Sood, who worked extensively on the COVID-19 problem in India, examined India's strategies against the COVID-19 pandemic.

Dr. Sood weaved together various elements that were crucial in India's successful strategies to address the COVID-19 pandemic. She shed light on several key factors that shaped India's approach, emphasizing the importance of intersectoral coordination and adopting a comprehensive, whole-government strategy (19).

By drawing on previous experiences, such as the annual vaccination of 26 million children, and integrating new strategies rooted in scientific evidence, such as leveraging technology to foster collaboration between urban and rural areas, fostering strong leadership, and encouraging societal participation, she shed light on how India managed to transform the pandemic into an endemic situation. The data indicates a significant decline in the transmission of the virus and a decrease in hospitalization rates. She said that it is crucial to remain vigilant and to take precautionary measures to safeguard against future pandemics (20).

Scan the QR Code or follow the link to listen
https://thepopmovement.org/podcast-public-health-uncoded/

What is COVID-19 and what are its Impacts on Health?

What is COVID-19 and what are its Impacts on Health?

COVID-19 is an infectious disease caused by the novel coronavirus SARS-CoV-2. It was first identified in December 2019 in Wuhan, China, and has since led to a global pandemic. The disease primarily spreads through respiratory droplets when an infected person coughs, sneezes, or talks. It can also spread by touching surfaces contaminated with the virus and then touching the face.

Key Impacts of COVID-19 on Health

Respiratory Symptoms:

- **Mild to Severe Illness**: Symptoms range from mild (fever, cough, fatigue) to severe (difficulty breathing, chest pain). Severe cases can lead to acute respiratory distress syndrome (ARDS), requiring hospitalization and ventilatory support.
- **Long-term Effects**: Some individuals experience long-lasting symptoms, known as "long COVID," which can include fatigue, shortness of breath, joint pain, and brain fog.

Systemic Effects:

- **Multisystem Inflammatory Syndrome**: In some cases, especially in children, COVID-19 can cause a severe inflammatory response affecting multiple organs (MIS-C).
- **Organ Damage**: The virus can cause damage to organs such as the heart, kidneys, liver, and brain, potentially leading to long-term health issues.

Impact on Vulnerable Populations:

- **Elderly and Pre-existing Conditions**: Older adults and individuals with underlying conditions (e.g., diabetes, heart disease, chronic respiratory disease) are at higher risk of severe illness and death.
- **Healthcare Disparities**: Marginalized communities often experience higher infection rates and worse health outcomes due to disparities in healthcare access and socio-economic factors.

Mental Health:

- **Psychological Stress**: The pandemic has caused widespread anxiety, depression, and stress due to illness fears, social isolation, and economic uncertainties.
- **Substance Abuse**: There has been an increase in substance abuse as individuals cope with the mental health impacts of the pandemic.

Impact on Healthcare Systems:

- **Strain on Healthcare Resources**: Hospitals and healthcare systems have been overwhelmed, leading to shortages of beds, medical supplies, and healthcare personnel.
- **Delayed Medical Care**: The focus on COVID-19 has led to delays in routine medical care, treatments, and surgeries, potentially worsening outcomes for non-COVID-related conditions.

Economic and Social Effects:

- **Economic Impact**: The pandemic has led to significant economic disruption, with job losses, business closures, and financial instability affecting millions of people.
- **Educational Disruption**: School closures and the shift to remote learning have impacted children's education and social development.

References

World Health Organization (WHO):

WHO provides comprehensive information on COVID-19, including its symptoms, transmission, and global impact. For more details, visit WHO's Coronavirus Disease (COVID-19) Page.

Centers for Disease Control and Prevention (CDC):

The CDC offers detailed guidance on COVID-19, including prevention, treatment, and the latest research on its health impacts. Learn more at CDC's COVID-19 Page.

National Institutes of Health (NIH):

NIH provides up-to-date research and information on the health impacts of COVID-19, including long-term effects and ongoing studies. Visit NIH's COVID-19 Page.

Johns Hopkins University & Medicine:

Johns Hopkins offers a COVID-19 resource center with data tracking, research updates, and expert insights on the pandemic's health impacts. Explore their resources at Johns Hopkins Coronavirus Resource Center.

The Lancet:

The Lancet publishes research articles and reviews on various aspects of COVID-19, including its health impacts and public health responses. Access their articles at The Lancet COVID-19 Resource Centre.

COVID-19 has had far-reaching impacts on global health, affecting physical health, mental wellbeing, healthcare systems, and socio-economic conditions. Addressing these impacts requires coordinated efforts in public health, healthcare provision, and social support systems.

PODCAST 13: PUBLIC HEALTH ENTREPRENEURSHIP

To address increasing public health challenges, an entrepreneurship approach must be employed to make an impact.

Nursing professionals need an entrepreneurial approach to working in government and private settings. This approach should aim to find innovative solutions to complex problems that organizations and individuals face. Using creative ways to solve problems and address health inequities is important.

This podcast discussion would be of interest to public health professionals, policy planners, and service providers.

Questions addressed

1. What does entrepreneurship mean?
2. How can entrepreneurship be operationalized within the programs?

Keywords

Bureaucracy, community health, entrepreneurship, intrapreneurship, partnership development, problem solving, and public health.

Quisha Umemba

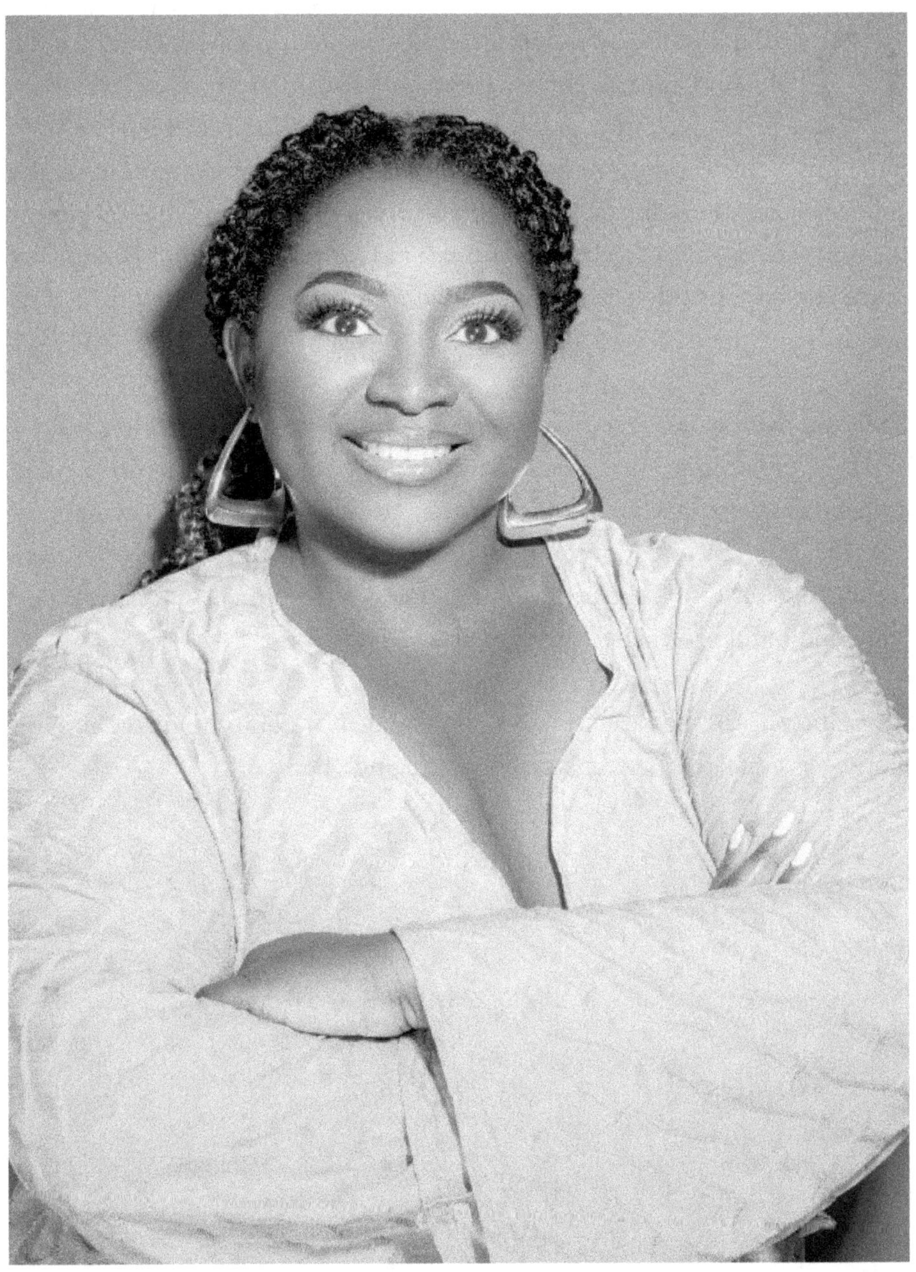

Quisha Umemba, CEO, Umemba Health

Quisha Umemba (pronounced "Kwee-shuh oooMEMbuh") is the CEO of Umemba Health, leveraging over 20 years of experience as a registered nurse, public health consultant, and entrepreneur. With numerous certifications, she has led various health initiatives and community collaborations. Her diverse roles include disaster response nurse leader for the American Red Cross, clinic coordinator for an endocrinology clinic, chief nurse at a local health department, and diabetes nurse consultant for a state health department.

Specializing in workforce training and development, Ms. Umemba designs and delivers unique curricula and training programs. Her methods blend conventional, experiential, and transformational approaches, earning her the title "The Trainer's Trainer." Additionally, as the principal of Quisha Umemba Consulting, she believes in "helping professionals" monetize their skills and build profitable consulting businesses.

A 3x author and passionate advocate for health equity, Quisha aims to empower, educate, and transform lives through her work.

Summary of the Podcast

In this podcast of Public Health Uncoded, Dr. Saroj Pachauri invited Ms. Quisha Umemba, a registered nurse and public health entrepreneur. Ms. Umemba shared her journey from bedside nursing to founding her public health consulting business, Umemba Health.

Ms. Umesha recounted her path to public health. She was not always a public health entrepreneur. She began her career as a registered nurse and later obtained a master's in public health (MPH). Witnessing the limitations of public health due to bureaucracy and funding restrictions, she decided to take a more solution-oriented approach.

She described her transition from bedside nursing to working with the Houston Health Department and later with the Texas Department of State Health Services. In these roles, she realized that working in government-funded public health systems had limitations. Bureaucracy, red tape, and reliance on grant funding hindered progress, innovation, and the ability to address community needs promptly. This frustration led her to consider starting her own business.

Ms. Quisha founded Umemba Health, a public health workforce development consulting and training agency. It addresses public health needs by developing curricula, toolkits, and training programs. She highlighted the importance of sustainability in public health initiatives aiming to empower communities to continue programs independently after initial funding ends.

Ms. Umemba described the concept of public health entrepreneurship as finding innovative solutions to problems faced by organizations or individuals. She distinguished this from the common perception of entrepreneurship involving venture capital and tech startups. She emphasized the role of problem-solving and creativity in addressing public health problems. She emphasized that public health professionals frequently act as "intrapreneurs" within their organizations, developing programs and initiatives to address health disparities. Ms. Umemba discussed the challenges and rewards of running her own business, highlighting the importance of being able to make both an impact and an income which is also covered in the book "Public Health Entrepreneurship: Navigating the Intersection of Purpose and Profit" authored by her. She encourages aspiring public health consultants to gain experience in traditional roles before venturing into entrepreneurship to develop problem-solving skills and practical knowledge (21).

Scan the QR Code or follow the link to listen
https://thepopmovement.org/podcast-public-health-uncoded/

What is public health entrepreneurship?

What is public health entrepreneurship?

Public Health Entrepreneurship involves applying innovative, business-oriented approaches to solve public health problems. It combines principles of public health with entrepreneurial practices to develop and implement solutions that can enhance health outcomes, improve healthcare delivery, and address social determinants of health. Public health entrepreneurs often work to bridge gaps in existing health systems, create new health technologies, or develop community-based initiatives.

Key Aspects of Public Health Entrepreneurship

Innovation in Health Solutions:

- Developing new products, services, or technologies that address public health challenges, such as wearable health monitors, mobile health apps, or telemedicine platforms.
- Creating innovative health programs and interventions that can be scaled to reach larger populations.

Social Impact:

- Focusing on creating sustainable and scalable solutions that improve the health and wellbeing of communities, particularly underserved populations.

- Addressing social determinants of health such as education, housing, and nutrition through community-based initiatives.

Business Models:

- Using sustainable business models that generate revenue while achieving public health goals. This can include social enterprises, non-profit organizations with earned income strategies, or hybrid models.
- Leveraging funding from various sources such as grants, investors, or public-private partnerships.

Policy and Advocacy:

- Engaging in policy advocacy to create supportive environments for public health innovations.
- Working with governments, NGOs, and other stakeholders to implement public health policies that facilitate entrepreneurial solutions.

Capacity Building:

- Training and mentoring health professionals and community leaders to develop entrepreneurial skills and approaches.
- Fostering a culture of innovation within public health institutions and organizations.

Examples of Public Health Entrepreneurship

Telehealth Platforms:

- Development of telehealth services to provide remote consultations and healthcare access, particularly in underserved areas.

Health Monitoring Devices:

- Creating affordable and user-friendly health monitoring devices for chronic diseases such as diabetes and hypertension.

Community Health Initiatives:

- Establishing community health programs that address local health needs, such as vaccination drives, nutrition education, and mental health support.

References

American Public Health Association (APHA):

APHA provides resources and articles on innovative approaches to public health, including entrepreneurship. Visit APHA's Innovation and Best Practices Page.

World Health Organization (WHO):

WHO offers resources on health innovation and entrepreneurship as part of its strategy to improve global health. Explore more at WHO's Health Innovation Page.

Harvard T.H. Chan School of Public Health:

Harvard provides courses and resources on public health entrepreneurship, emphasizing the importance of innovation in solving health challenges. Learn more at Harvard's Public Health Entrepreneurship Page.

Global Health Delivery Online (GHDonline):

GHDonline is a platform that connects health professionals and entrepreneurs to share ideas and solutions for global health challenges. Visit GHDonline.

Journal of Public Health Management and Practice:

This journal publishes research and case studies on public health entrepreneurship and innovation. Access their articles at Journal of Public Health Management and Practice.

Public health entrepreneurship is a dynamic and growing field that leverages innovation and business strategies to tackle some of the most pressing health issues facing communities worldwide.

PODCAST 14: NAVIGATING THE INTERSECTION OF WATER, CLIMATE AND PRIMARY HEALTHCARE

Water, climate change, and primary healthcare are all important for improving health. These interventions are, however, currently implemented in siloes. It is important to integrate these interventions to address health problems holistically.

Climate change is a public health crisis that impacts physical and mental health and wellbeing. Thus far, programs have not addressed mental health problems, which are increasing significantly in today's world.

There is an urgent need to design programs and formulate policies for holistically addressing human health. Empowering people and fostering community engagement to ensure accountability is also important. Technology and innovation must be leveraged to address these intersected issues effectively.

The audience for this podcast discussion includes public health professionals, researchers, policy planners, and service providers.

Questions addressed

1. What is the importance of understanding the intersection of water,

climate change, and primary healthcare? What measures can be undertaken to address these problems?

2. How can communities be empowered so that they demand services?

3. What measures/ call to action need to be undertaken to address the intersection?

4. What is the significance of primary healthcare systems as the fulcrum for bringing these intersections together.

Keywords

Climate change, primary healthcare, vector-borne diseases, mental health, water and sanitation, water security, and community empowerment

Debadutta Parija

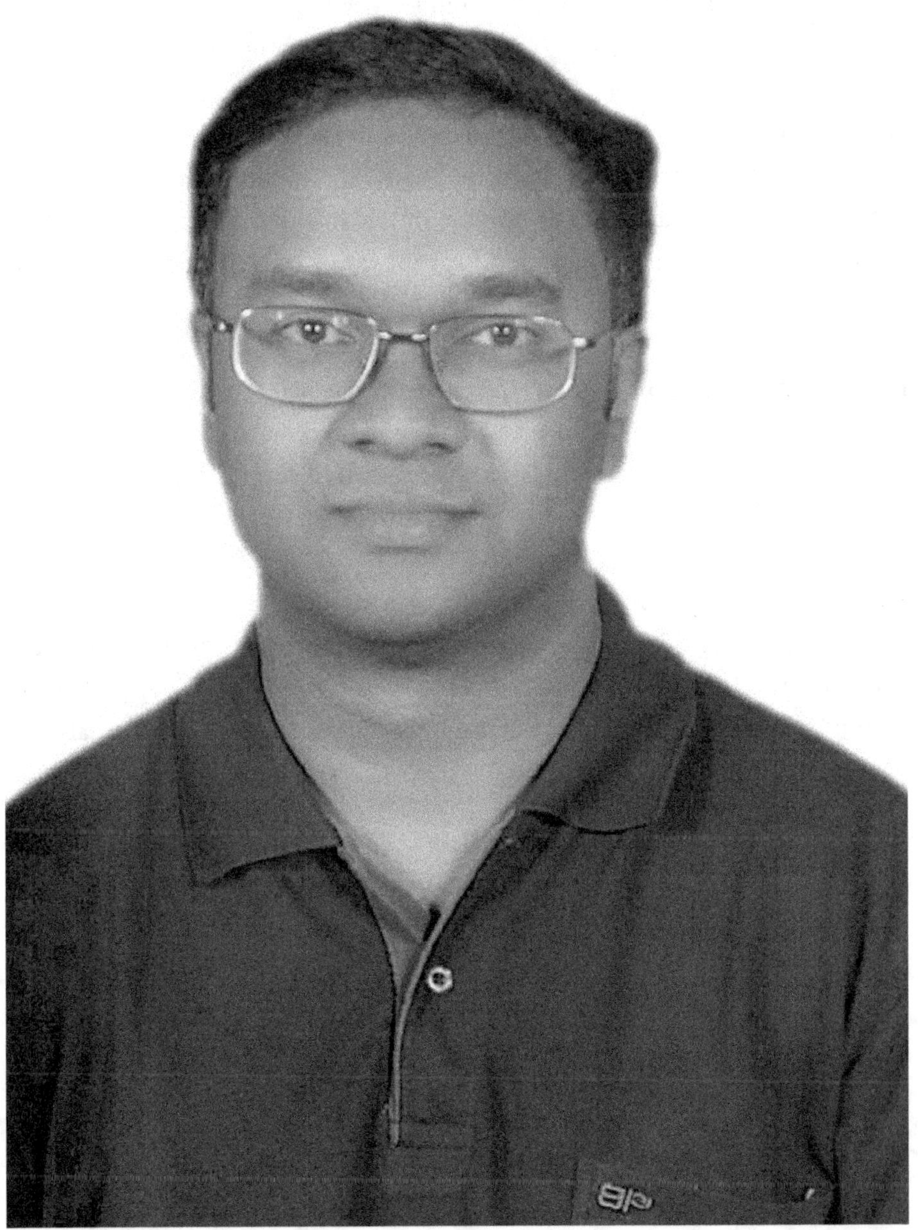

Dr. Debadutta Parija, Country Lead for TB, Infectious Diseases and Surveillance, NISHTHA, Jhpiego, India

Dr. Debadutta Parija is the Country Lead for TB, Infectious Diseases, and Surveillance at NISHTHA, Jhpiego, India. He holds an MBBS from Srirama Chandra Bhanja Medical College, Cuttack, Odisha, and an MBA in health systems. With over twenty years of experience in national health programs, Dr. Parija has worked in senior management roles with the government and international public health organizations such as WHO, Jhpiego, and the Foundation for Innovative New Diagnostics (FIND).

His expertise spans health systems strengthening, TB control, TB diagnostics management, and family planning. Dr. Parija has extensive experience engaging with donors, writing grant proposals, and managing multi-million-dollar projects. He has served as a WHO consultant supporting TB programs internationally.

A technical expert, Dr. Parija has contributed to national committees for developing guidelines on TB, multidrug-resistant tuberculosis and extensively drug-resistant tuberculosis MDR/XDR-TB, HIV-TB, pediatric TB, and extra-pulmonary TB. He has numerous publications in international peer-reviewed journals.

Summary of the podcast

In this podcast of Public Health Uncoded, Dr. Saroj Pachauri and the expert Dr. Debadutta Parija discussed the crucial intersection of water, climate, and primary healthcare. Dr. Parija highlighted the traditional siloed approach to these problems and emphasized the need to implement integrated programs. He pointed out that water is a fundamental determinant of health, affecting everything from sanitation to disease transmission, and that climate change exacerbates existing water-related challenges, introducing new health risks and altering disease patterns.

Dr. Pachauri reflected on past efforts to integrate health services like family planning and reproductive health, noting that strong advocacy was crucial for success. Dr. Pachauri and Dr Parija, both agreed that empowering communities to demand services and hold systems accountable is vital. Dr. Parija mentioned initiatives in India, such as the formation of community wellness committees, which are starting to ask pertinent questions to health departments, fostering accountability and better service delivery.

The conversation shifted to the importance of mental health, which is often neglected and stigmatized. Dr. Parija stressed the need to raise awareness and capacitate primary healthcare providers to address mental health issues, which are increasingly intertwined with other health conditions and are exacerbated by climate change.

As Dr. Parija concluded, he underscored the need for policy-level resilience and adaptation strategies, community engagement, and the need to document successful initiatives to serve as models for other regions. He advocated for leveraging technology and innovation to address these interconnected issues effectively.

Scan the QR Code or follow the link to listen
https://thepopmovement.org/podcast-public-health-uncoded/

What are the intersections between water, climate, and primary healthcare?

What are the intersections between water, climate, and primary healthcare?

The intersection between water, climate, and primary healthcare is crucial for ensuring the wellbeing of populations, particularly in the context of climate change. Access to clean water, climate change impacts, and primary healthcare effectiveness are deeply interconnected and have significant implications for public health.

Key Intersections

Water and Primary Healthcare:

- **Clean Water and Sanitation**: Access to clean water and proper sanitation is essential for preventing waterborne diseases such as cholera, dysentery, and typhoid. Primary healthcare systems are critical in providing education, resources, and treatment for these diseases.
- **Hygiene Practices**: Primary healthcare facilities must maintain high hygiene standards to prevent infections. Adequate water supply is necessary for handwashing, cleaning, and sterilizing medical equipment.

Climate Change and Water Resources:

- **Water Scarcity**: Climate change leads to altered precipitation patterns, causing droughts and water shortages in many regions. This affects the availability of clean water for drinking, agriculture, and sanitation.
- **Flooding and Contamination**: Increased frequency and severity of flooding can contaminate water supplies with pollutants and pathogens, leading to outbreaks of waterborne diseases.

Climate Change and Primary Healthcare:

- **Health Impacts**: Climate change exacerbates health issues such as heat-related illnesses, respiratory problems from poor air quality, and the spread of vector-borne diseases like malaria and dengue fever. Primary healthcare systems need to adapt to these emerging health threats.
- **Infrastructure Resilience**: Primary healthcare facilities must be resilient to extreme weather events. This includes ensuring that buildings can withstand storms and that there are contingency plans for maintaining healthcare services during disasters.

Integrated Approaches:

- **Water Management**: Sustainable water management practices can mitigate the impacts of climate change and ensure a reliable water supply for primary healthcare facilities.
- **Community Health Programs**: Integrating climate and water considerations into community health programs can improve overall health outcomes. For example, educating communities about water conservation, climate adaptation strategies, and preventive health measures can enhance resilience.

References

World Health Organization (WHO):

WHO provides resources on the links between climate change, water, and health, including strategies for integrating these elements into healthcare planning. For more details, visit WHO's Climate Change and Health Page and WHO's Water Sanitation and Health Page.

Centers for Disease Control and Prevention (CDC):

The CDC offers information on climate effects on health and the importance of water, sanitation, and hygiene (WASH) in healthcare settings. Learn more at CDC's Climate and Health Page and CDC's WASH Page.

United Nations Children's Fund (UNICEF):

UNICEF works on improving access to clean water and sanitation as part of its mission to enhance children's health, emphasizing the impacts of climate change. Visit UNICEF's Water, Sanitation and Hygiene (WASH) Page and UNICEF's Climate Change Page.

Intergovernmental Panel on Climate Change (IPCC):

The IPCC provides comprehensive reports on the impacts of climate change, including those on water resources and health. Access their reports at IPCC's Reports Page.

Global Water Partnership (GWP):

GWP offers resources and research on integrated water resources management, emphasizing the need to address climate change and health together. Explore more at GWP's Climate Change Page.

Understanding the intersection of water, climate, and primary healthcare is essential for developing comprehensive strategies that promote sustainable health outcomes and resilience in the face of climate change.

AUTHORS' BIOS

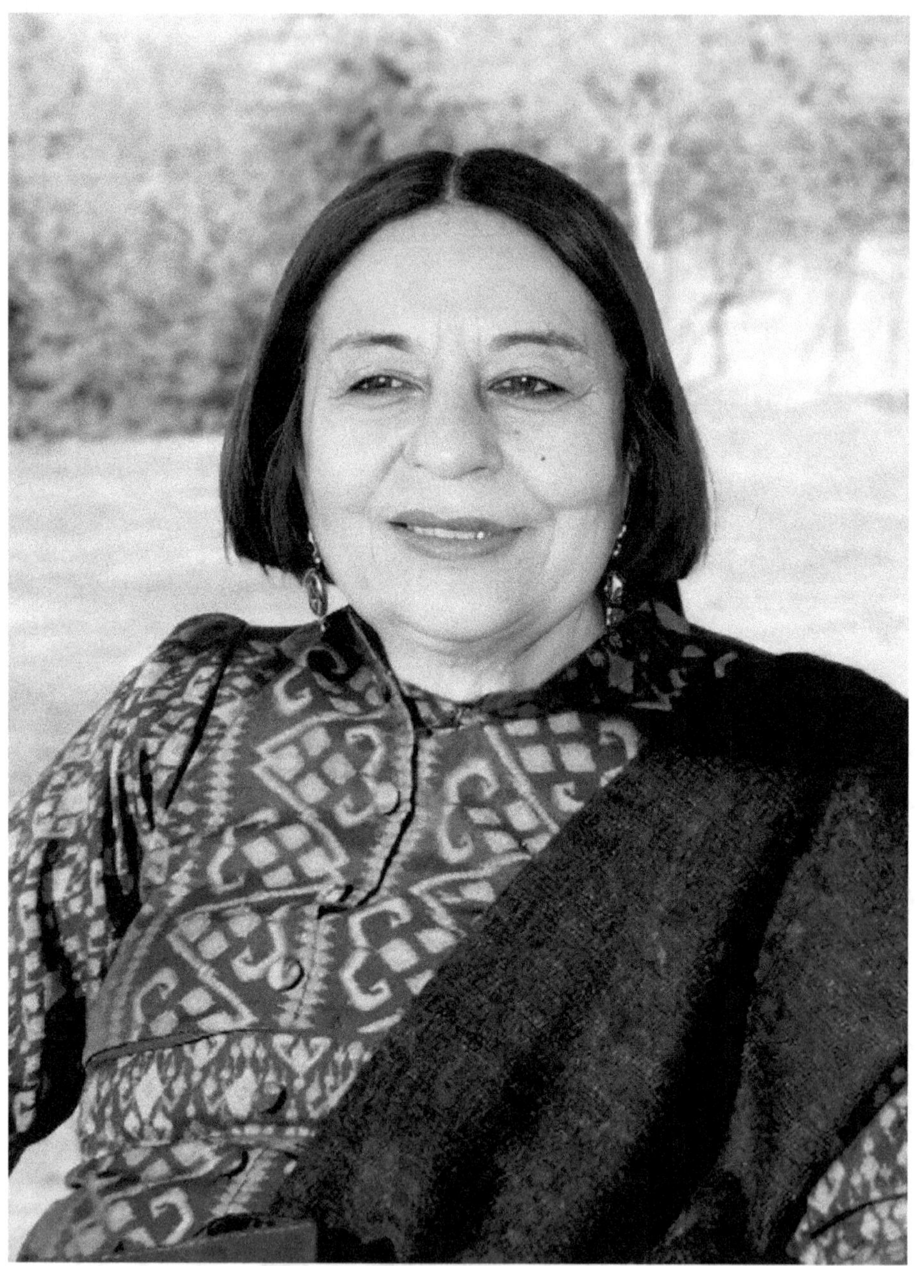

Dr. Saroj Pachauri

Dr. Saroj Pachauri, Public Health Specialist, Trustee, Center for Human Progress, New Delhi, India, and Director, the POP (Protect Our Planet) Movement, New York, USA

As a public health physician, Dr. Pachauri has been extensively engaged with research on family planning, maternal and child health, sexual and reproductive health and rights, HIV and AIDS, and poverty, gender and youth. In 1996, she joined as Regional Director, South and East Asia, Population Council and established its regional office in New Delhi which she managed until 2014. In 2011, she was awarded the prestigious title of Distinguished Scholar, an honor rarely bestowed.

She worked with the Ford Foundation's New Delhi Office (1983-1994) and supported child survival, women's health, sexual and reproductive health, and HIV and AIDS programs. Before that, she worked with the International Fertility Research Program (IFRP) which was later renamed Family Health International (1971-1975) and the India Fertility Research Program (1975-1983). She designed and monitored multi-centric clinical trials globally to assess the safety and effectiveness of fertility control technologies. During 1962-1971, as faculty of the Departments of Preventive and Social Medicine at the Lady Hardinge Medical College, New Delhi and the Institute of Medicine Sciences, Varanasi, she helped to develop this new discipline.

She has published twelve books and contributed chapters to 20 books. She has over 100 publications in peer-reviewed journals and several articles in print media.

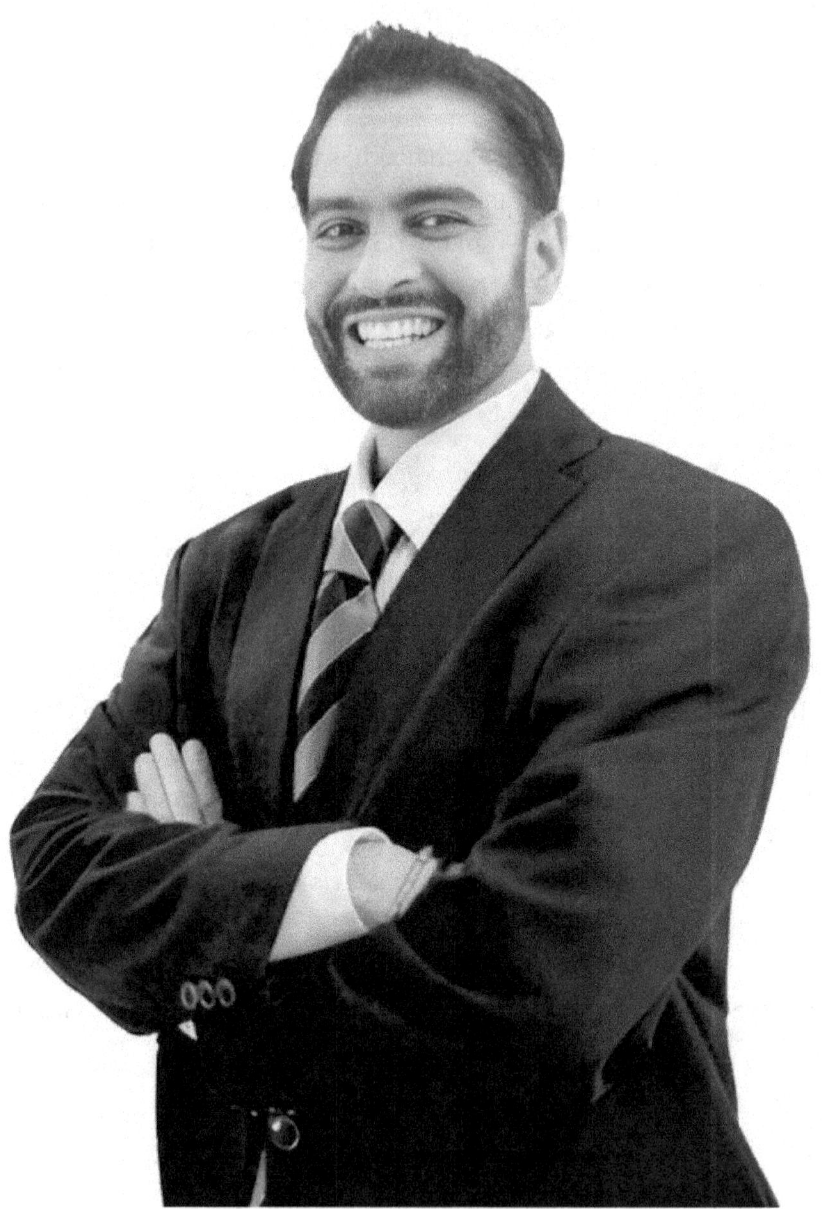

Dr. Ash Pachauri, PhD

Dr. Ash Pachauri has a PhD in behavioral science and technology and a master's in international management. Having worked with McKinsey & Company before pursuing a career in the social development arena, Dr. Pachauri's experience in public health and sustainable development emerges from a range of initiatives. Notably, he has made significant contributions to the Bill & Melinda Gates Foundation by contributing to its public health and community agenda, the UN by focusing on youth, health, and the Sustainable Development Goals (SDGs), and the Center for Disease Control program interventions in the US by focusing on community interventions, especially for vulnerable youth. He has also been instrumental in founding and building the POP Movement and the World Sustainable Development Forum. He is a technical adviser to the World Health Organization on Self-Care Global Guidelines to support youth, communities, and global governments.

Dr. Pachauri has been a pioneer in the use of information technology for development. His innovative approaches have been key to spearheading community- and youth-led self-care interventions, leading to global capacity building and adoption of self-care among youth. As a master trainer in behavior change communications and strategic leadership, Dr. Pachauri has led over 20,000 workshops, events, and global outreach to youth and communities to promote global health and climate action.

Widely published, winner of the prestigious Overseas Research Scholarship, awarded for advanced studies in the U.K., and recognized for his academic achievements, Dr. Pachauri's awards and recognitions reflect his significant contributions to the field. The United Nations has recognized Dr. Pachauri for his dedication and leadership in their flagship publication, "Portraits of Commitment," A testament to his influence in the field. In 2021, he was awarded the GlobalMindED Inclusive Leadership Award for action in Energy and Sustainability, a recognition of his commitment to inclusive and sustainable development among young people worldwide. He is an Associate Fellow of the World Academy of Art and Science, a position that underscores his academic standing. Dr. Pachauri serves on the Boards and Advisory groups of several organizations and initiatives worldwide, including the global movement on bone health, the Climate Change Coalition, and the Global Union of Scientists for Peace. He demonstrates leadership and influence in the global health and climate action community.

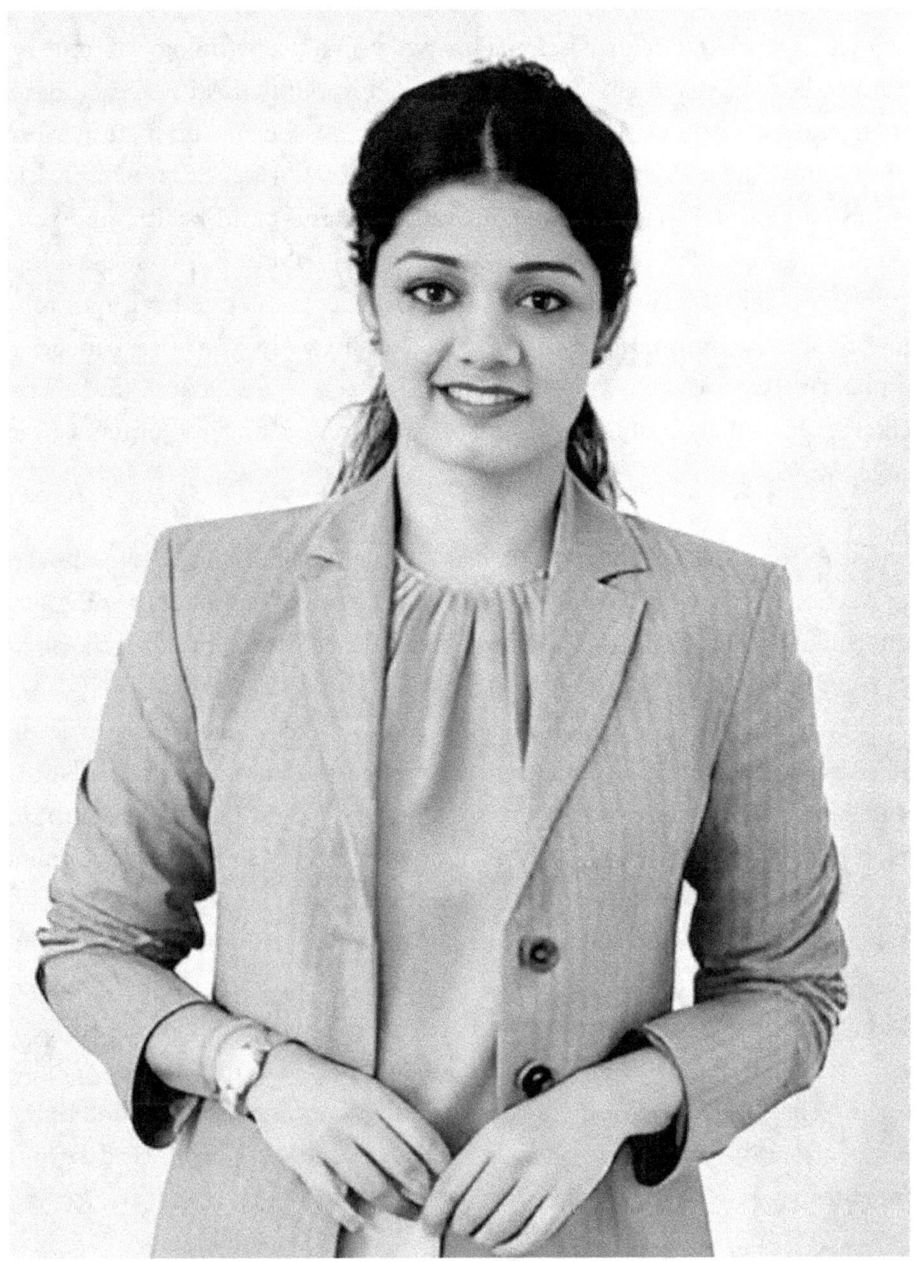

Drishya Pathak

Drishya Pathak obtained a master's in public health (MPH) in 2019. She worked as a healthcare professional for two years in a pathology laboratory. For the last six years, she has been engaged in public health and climate change. In this period, she worked as a research associate and mentor with the POP (Protect Our Planet) Movement. She worked on public health issues like COVID-19, tuberculosis, maternal and child health, and self-care for sexual and reproductive health. Her contributions include leading studies on self-care practices for sexual and reproductive health among marginalized communities and youth. Additionally, she spearheaded a pioneering investigation into the health impacts of sargassum (linked to changes in climatic conditions) on coastal communities in Quintana Roo state, Mexico.

She was honored with the prestigious Alexander Von Humboldt Climate Protection Fellowship 2023 in Germany for a project on understanding the interlinkages between climate change, biodiversity loss, and human health.

With a strong focus on public health, Ms. Pathak played a key role in various projects. She presented several publications and reports, including on Universal Health Coverage, Civil Society and Community Consultation, WHO Self-Care Guidelines dissemination, Joint United Nations Program on HIV/AIDS (UNAIDS), and Asia Pacific Council of AIDS Service Organizations (APCASO) Youth Consultation on Sustainable Development Goals. She successfully implemented the project Medication Event Reminder Monitor (MERM) Deployment for Tuberculosis which was jointly funded by Bill & Melinda Gates Foundation's (BMGF's) and United States Agency for International Development (USAID). She worked with the Nada India Foundation (NIF) addressing health, child and adolescent rights, and a drug-free lifestyle.

As a POP Youth Mentor with the POP Movement, she has played a pivotal role in global community-led projects focused on climate mitigation and adaptation. She collaborates closely with youth leaders in different countries and recently planted 5,000 trees in India.

She has contributed chapters to five books and has co-authored five research articles, reflecting her dedication to advancing knowledge and generating evidence.

LIST OF ACRONYMS

This list of acronyms (see below) provides easy access for our readers.

AIDS - Acquired Immunodeficiency Syndrome

APCASO - Asia Pacific Council of AIDS Service Organizations

BMGF - Bill & Melinda Gates Foundation

CEDPA - Centre for Development and Population Activities

EDCs - Endocrine Disrupting Chemicals

FIND - Foundation for Innovative New Diagnostics

HIV - Human Immunodeficiency Virus

IAVI - International AIDS Vaccine Initiative

IFRP - International Fertility Research Program

IPN - Instituto Politecnico Nacional

IRB - Institutional Review Board

IUDs - Intra-Uterine Devices

MDR/XDR-TB - Multidrug-Resistant/Extensively Drug-Resistant Tuberculosis

MERM - Medication Event Reminder Monitor

NCDs - Non-Communicable Diseases

NGO - Non-Governmental Organization

NIF - Nada India Foundation

NITI Aayog - National Institution for Transforming India

PATH - Program for Appropriate Technology in Health

POPs - Persistent Organic Pollutants

POP Movement - (Protect Our Planet) Movement

PrEP - Pre-exposure Prophylaxis

RTI - Reproductive Tract Infections

SDG - Sustainable Development Goal

SIDA - Swedish International Development Authority

SRHR - Sexual and Reproductive Health and Rights

TB - Tuberculosis

UNAIDS - Joint United Nations Programme on HIV/AIDS

USAID - United States Agency for International Development

RESOURCE LIST

Definitions of terms

Sexual health: The World Health Organization defines sexual health as a state of physical, emotional, mental and social wellbeing related to sexuality; it is not merely the absence of disease, dysfunction or infirmity.

Maternal mortality: The annual number of female deaths from any cause related to or aggravated by pregnancy or its management (excluding accidental or incidental causes) during pregnancy and childbirth or within 42 days of termination of pregnancy, irrespective of the duration and site of the pregnancy.

Morbidity: Is the state of being symptomatic or unhealthy for a disease or condition.

Maternal health: Maternal health refers to the health of women during pregnancy, childbirth, and the postnatal period.

Family planning: The ability of individuals and couples to anticipate and attain their desired number of children and the spacing and timing of their births.

Intra-uterine devices (IUDs): An intrauterine device (IUD) is a long-term contraception method.

Abortion: The World Health Organization (WHO) define abortion as pregnancy termination prior to 20 weeks' gestation or a fetus born weighing less than 500 g. Despite this, definitions vary widely according to state laws."

HIV/AIDS: Human immunodeficiency virus (HIV) is an infection that attacks the body's immune system. Acquired immunodeficiency syndrome (AIDS) is the most advanced stage of the disease.

Pre-exposure prophylaxis (PrEP): Pre-exposure prophylaxis or "PrEP" is the use of an antiretroviral medication by HIV-negative people to reduce the risk of HIV acquisition.

Reproductive tract infections (RTIs): RTIs are defined as any infection of the reproductive system. They include STIs and other infections of the reproductive system that are not caused by sexual contact.

Sexually transmitted infections: STIs are infections transmitted from person to person by sexual contact.

Gender: Gender refers to the characteristics of women, men, girls and boys that are socially constructed. This includes norms, behaviors and roles associated with being a woman, man, girl or boy, as well as relationships with each other. As a social construct, gender varies from society to society and can change over time.

Determinants of health: The determinants of health include: the social and economic environment, the physical environment, and. the person's individual characteristics and behaviors.

Public health policy: Public health policy is defined as the laws, regulations, actions, and decisions implemented within society in order to promote wellness and ensure that specific health goals are met.

Global health: Global health is an area for study, research, and practice that places a priority on improving health and achieving equity in health for all people worldwide.

Bioethics: Bioethics is the study of ethical, social, and legal issues that arise in biomedicine and biomedical research.

Communicable diseases: Communicable or infectious diseases are caused by microorganisms such as bacteria, viruses, parasites and fungi that can be spread, directly or indirectly, from one person to another.

Non-communicable diseases: The term non-communicable diseases (NCDs) refers to a group of conditions that are not mainly caused by an acute infection, result in long-term health consequences and often create a need for long-term treatment and care. These conditions include cancers, cardiovascular disease, diabetes, and chronic lung illnesses.

Antiretroviral therapy: Antiretroviral therapy (ART) is treatment of people infected with human immunodeficiency virus (HIV) using anti-HIV drugs

Misinformation: Misinformation is false or inaccurate information—getting the facts wrong.

Disinformation: Disinformation is false information which is deliberately intended to mislead—intentionally misstating the facts.

Podcast links

Public Health Uncoded: Link to the podcast webpage https://thepopmove
ment.org/podcast-public-health-uncoded/

Public Health Uncoded: Link to the podcast YouTube channel https://www.
youtube.com/playlist?list=PLh7T-_ypS9Isy0XPt06v6CrCsycmqjuKj

Public Health Uncoded: Link to the podcast Spotify channel https://open.s
potify.com/show/0dP2B9mSgcqTNRf80DnT7B?si=74d93b470f5e4237

Websites

POP (Protect Our Planet) Movement www.thepopmovement.org

Rotary Action Group https://rotaryrmch.org/member/8121df5b-552c-11
e7-bafc-f04da27538fb

Centre for Catalyzing Change https://www.c3india.org/

Gynuity Health Projects https://gynuity.org/

HIV/AIDS Alliance https://allianceindia.org/

Swedish International Development Authority https://www.sida.se/en

International Planned Parenthood Federation https://www.ippf.org/

Global Health Strategies https://globalhealthstrategies.com/

International AIDS Vaccine Initiative https://www.iavi.org/

Editorji https://www.editorji.com/

FXB Climate Advocates https://www.fxbclimateadvocates.org/

Universidad Nacional Autónoma de México https://www.unam.mx/

Instituto Politecnico Nacional (IPN) https://www.ipn.mx/ingles/

Mu Gamma Consultants https://www.mugammaconsultants.com/

Jhpiego-India https://www.jhpiego.org/countries-we-support/india/

Centre for Development and Population Activities (CEDPA) part of Plan International https://plan-international.org/

Umemba Health https://www.umembahealth.com/

Foundation for Innovative New Diagnostics (FIND) https://www.finddx.org/

REFERENCES

The following list of references ensures easy reading for our audience.

Townsend J, Sitruk-Ware R, RamaRao S & Sailer J. Contraceptive technologies for global health: Ethically getting to safe, effective and acceptable options for women and men. Drug Delivery and Translational Research. 2020 Mar 2; 10(2).

Speidel J, Townsend J, Williams E, Quam J & Thompson K. Commentary on research to improve contraceptive and multipurpose prevention technologies. Contraception. 2020 Jan 6; 101(3): 148-152.

Gogoi A, Joshi M. Claiming as equals: journey of women leaders. In: Pachauri S, Verma RK, editors. Transforming unequal gender relations in India and beyond: An intersectional perspective on challenges and opportunities. Springer Nature. 2023 Sep 09: 169–182.

Gogoi A, Ravi T. Respectful Maternity Care: A Cornerstone for Improving Maternal Health. In: Pachauri S, Verma RK, editors. Transforming unequal gender relations in India and beyond: An intersectional perspective on challenges and opportunities. Springer Nature. 2023 Sep 09: 229-237.

Stanton M, Gogoi A. Dignity and respect in maternity care. British Medical Journal. 2022 Mar 1; 5.

Gogoi A, Manoranjini M & Banerjee R. The impact of COVID-19 on adolescents, nodal teachers, and frontline workers. In: Pachauri S, Pachauri A, editors. Global perspectives of COVID-19 pandemic on health, education, and role of media. Springer Nature. 2023 Aug 15: 233-247.

Winikoff B & Sheldon W. Use of Medicines Changing the Face of Abortion. International Perspectives on Sexual and Reproductive Health. 2012 Sep 6; 38: 164.

Winikoff B, Ellertson C, Elul B & Sivin I. Acceptability and feasibility of early pregnancy termination by mifepristone-misoprostol. Results of a large multicenter trial in the United States. Mifepristone Clinical Trials Group. Archives of Family Medicine. 1998; 7(4): 360–366.

Joint United Nations Programme on HIV/AIDS. The path that ends Aids: 2023 UNAIDS - Global Report 2023. Joint United Nations Programme on HIV/AIDS. 2023 Jul 13.

Nath MB. Gender insights into a unique threat to human development. In: Pachauri S, Pachauri A, editors. Health dimensions of COVID-19 in India and beyond. Springer Nature; 2022 Apr: 227–243.

Nath MB. The costs of ignoring gender. In: Pachauri S, Verma RK, editors. Transforming unequal gender relations in India and beyond: An intersectional perspective on challenges and opportunities. Springer Nature; 2023 Sep 9: 389–404.

Nayyar A, Bose N, Shrivastava R, Basu R & Andries S. Social media in the time of a pandemic. In: Pachauri S, Pachauri A, editors. Global perspectives of COVID-19 pandemic on health, education, and role of media. Springer Nature. 2023 Aug 15: 289–303.

Weinstein K. Gender and climate change: Maximizing women's potential to lead on climate mitigation and adaptation. In: Pachauri S, Verma RK, editors. Transforming Unequal Gender Relations in India and Beyond: An Intersectional Perspective on Challenges and Opportunities. Springer Nature. 2023: 183–193.

Vega H, Tamayo L, Cervantes-Jimenez M, Sarmiento G A. Epistemologia-y-Pedagogia-climatica-en-Mexico. 2022 Jun 26.

Sevilla N, Urias D, Rodriguez S.P & Acuna E.M. Massive presence of sargassum on the coasts of Quintana Roo, Mexico and its relationship with human health and air quality. In: Pachauri S, Pachauri A, Jonathan M.P, editors. Health and climate change: Unraveling the connections. Elsevier. 2024 Sep (*In process*).

Mohapatra P, Bharat G, Roy Basu A & Adams H. Regulatory framework, policies, and programs in POPs Management in India. In 2023: 19–39.

Chakraborty P, Chandra J S, Roy Basu A & Bharat G. An Indian perspective on sources of persistent organic pollutants associated with plastic handling: Consequences of COVID-19 pandemic. In: Chakraborty P, Bharat G, Sinha S, editors. Managing persistent organic pollutants in India. Springer Nature. 2023 Jul: 41–61.

Sharma BM, Scheringer M, Chakraborty P, Bharat G, Steindal E, Trasande L, et al. Unlocking India's potential in managing Endocrine-Disrupting Chemicals (EDCs): Importance, challenges, and opportunities. Exposure and Health. 2022 Dec 12;15(4).

Sood B, Srivastava VK & Mohanty N. Addressing the urgency and magnitude of the COVID-19 pandemic in India by improving healthcare workforce resilience. In: Pachauri S, Pachauri A, editors. Global perspectives of covid-19 pandemic on health, education, and role. Springer Nature; 2023 Aug 15: 25–44.

REFERENCES

Sood B. Investing in a resilient and responsive healthcare system during COVID-19 pandemic. In: Pachauri S, Pachauri A, editors. Health dimensions of COVID-19 in India and beyond. Springer Nature. 2022 Apr: 27–52.

Umemba Q. Public health entrepreneurship: Navigating the intersection of purpose and profit.

If you find this book helpful, we would appreciate it if you left us a favorable review!

48653CB00004BA/1344